Tissue Adhesives in Clinical Medicine

Second Edition

James V. Quinn, MD, MS

Department of Surgery
Stanford University
Palo Alto, California

2005
BC Decker Inc
Hamilton

BC Decker Inc
P.O. Box 620, L.C.D. 1
Hamilton, Ontario L8N 3K7
Tel: 905-522-7017; 800-568-7281
Fax: 905-522-7839; 888-311-4987
E-mail: info@bcdecker.com
www.bcdecker.com

BC Decker

05 06 07 08 / WPC / 9 8 7 6 5 4 3 2 1
Printed in the United States of America
ISBN 1-55009-282-0

Sales and Distribution

United States
BC Decker Inc
P.O. Box 785
Lewiston, NY 14092-0785
Tel: 905-522-7017; 800-568-7281
Fax: 905-522-7839; 888-311-4987
E-mail: info@bcdecker.com
www.bcdecker.com

Canada
BC Decker Inc
20 Hughson Street South
P.O. Box 620, LCD 1
Hamilton, Ontario L8N 3K7
Tel: 905-522-7017; 800-568-7281
Fax: 905-522-7839; 888-311-4987
E-mail: info@bcdecker.com
www.bcdecker.com

Foreign Rights
John Scott & Company
International Publishers' Agency
P.O. Box 878
Kimberton, PA 19442
Tel: 610-827-1640
Fax: 610-827-1671
E-mail: jsco@voicenet.com

Japan
Igaku-Shoin Ltd.
Foreign Publications Department
3-24-17 Hongo
Bunkyo-ku, Tokyo, Japan 113-8719
Tel: 3 3817 5680
Fax: 3 3815 6776
E-mail: fd@igaku-shoin.co.jp

UK, Europe, Scandinavia, Middle East
Elsevier Science
Customer Service Department
Foots Cray High Street
Sidcup, Kent
DA14 5HP, UK
Tel: 44 (0) 208 308 5760
Fax: 44 (0) 181 308 5702
E-mail: cservice@harcourt.com

Singapore, Malaysia,Thailand, Philippines, Indonesia, Vietnam, Pacific Rim, Korea
Elsevier Science Asia
583 Orchard Road
#09/01, Forum
Singapore 238884
Tel: 65-737-3593
Fax: 65-753-2145

Australia, New Zealand
Elsevier Science Australia
Customer Service Department
STM Division
Locked Bag 16
St. Peters, New South Wales, 2044
Australia
Tel: 61 02 9517-8999
Fax: 61 02 9517-2249
E-mail: stmp@harcourt.com.au
www.harcourt.com.au

Mexico and Central America
ETM SA de CV
Calle de Tula 59
Colonia Condesa
06140 Mexico DF, Mexico
Tel: 52-5-5553-6657
Fax: 52-5-5211-8468
E-mail:
editoresdetextosmex@prodigy.net.mx

Brazil
Tecmedd
Av. Maurílio Biagi, 2850
City Ribeirão Preto – SP – CEP: 14021-000
Tel: 0800 992236
Fax: (16) 3993-9000
E-mail: tecmedd@tecmedd.com.br

India, Bangladesh, Pakistan, Sri Lanka
Elsevier Health Sciences Division
Customer Service Department
17A/1, Main Ring Road
Lajpat Nagar IV
New Delhi – 110024, India
Tel: 91 11 2644 7160-64
Fax: 91 11 2644 7156
E-mail: esindia@vsnl.net

Contents

Preface

It has been over 6 years since the publication of *Tissue Adhesives in Wound Care,* which coincided with the approval of the first cyanoacrylate tissue adhesive by the Food and Drug Administration (FDA) in the United States. It was a small book or monograph written primarily as an educational tool for physicians on how to properly use the product known as Dermabond (Ethicon Inc., Somerville, NJ). As the first cyanoacrylate tissue adhesive approved for wound closure, it was a great breakthrough. However, "gluing a wound" somehow had a connotation that it was easy and required little skill or knowledge to use in place of suturing, a skill in which most physicians and surgeons have spent years developing expertise. People who use tissue adhesives and read our text realize that tissue adhesives are not without limitations and require skill and education to use them properly. We hoped that our initial edition served its purpose and helped providers learn how to appropriately select wounds and apply tissue adhesives properly for wound closure.

Since our original work, other cyanoacrylate adhesives have been approved for wound closure and multiple other uses. Non-cyanoacrylate adhesives, such as fibrin-based adhesives and other synthetic and protein polymers, have become more popular and deserve attention, as do cements. Our new edition is broader in scope and depth and includes all types of tissue adhesives, their proper indications, and their uses. Our goal is to have a book that is an in-depth reference on all tissue adhesives so that physicians and surgeons have one place to look to learn about the various materials, their indications, and how to use them properly. To achieve this goal, I solicited the help of expert colleagues, and we put together a book that is a practical and in-depth guide.

Most chapters follow a similar format, looking at the history and development, chemistry, toxicity, clinical use, regulation, cost, effectiveness, and optimal application techniques. Potential pitfalls are identified, as are practical tips to achieve optimal outcomes. Figures have been used to help illustrate points, and, where possible, video files are incorporated onto the accompanying compact disc. My colleagues at the FDA have contributed a chapter on the regulation of tissue adhesives so that one can understand the availability and regulation around these products. All chapters are appropriately referenced for those wishing to explore the literature in more detail.

I feel that we have achieved our goal to provide readers with an in-depth practical guide to all tissue adhesives used in clinical medicine and trust that those who read it will find it useful.

James V. Quinn, MD, MS
Stanford, California
December 2004

Contributors

Sandra G. Burks, BSN
Department of Surgery
University of Virginia
Charlottesville, Virginia

George J. Mattamal, PhD
Division of General, Restorative, and Neurological Devices
Office of Device Evaluation
Center for Devices and Radiological Health
US Food and Drug Administration
Rockville, Maryland

Jennifer L. Maw, MD, FRCS
Department of Otolaryngology
Stanford University
Stanford, California

Roshan Prabhu, BS
Department of Surgery
University of Florida
Gainesville, Florida

K. Ümit Yüksel, PhD
CryoLife, Inc
Kennesaw, Georgia

James V. Quinn, MD, MS
Department of Surgery
Stanford University
Palo Alto, California

CDR Stephen P. Rhodes, USPHS
Division of General, Restorative and Neurological Devices
Office of Device Evaluation
Center for Devices and Radiological Health
US Food and Drug Administration
Rockville, Maryland

William D. Spotnitz, MD
Department of Surgery
University of Virginia
Charlottesville, Virginia

1 Overview of Tissue Adhesives

James V. Quinn, MD, MS

Historical Perspective

Interest in treating wounds and stopping hemorrhage can be dated back to our ancestors, *Australopithecus africans*. As violence and war appeared in their culture, they needed to deal with wounds. There is evidence that more than a million years ago, these ancestors made attempts to deal with open wounds, bleeding, and infection with simple dressings using grass and leaves.[1] The first suturing of wounds by primitive people may be older than that done by *Homo sapiens*. Primitive people closed wounds by sewing them together with muscle fibers or shreds of tendon. They closed large wounds by inserting spikes along the edges of the wounds and then tying them together with cloth or hide. The oldest suture dates back to a twenty-first Dynasty mummy in approximately 1100 BC (Figure 1–1). It is evident that there was a delay before suturing became the standard wound closure. It was made popular only by the Egyptians, ancient Greeks, and Indians. Historians believe that early man recognized that sutures were a mixed blessing, at times causing infection and preventing wound healing. Early people looked for alternatives to thread and needle. The use of adhesive tapes and gum adhesives from plants can be dated back 4,000 years. The use of skin clips can be attributed to early cultures that used the jaws of ants to approximate wound edges (Figure 1–2). Modern people have continued to refine the suture to its current status, but the search for alternative methods and devices for wound closure continues to evolve.[1,2]

Over time, sutures have become the standard of wound closure. Cur-

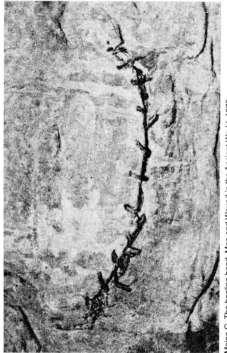

Majno G. The healing hand. Man and Wound in the Ancient World. 1975.

■ **FIGURE 1–1** Sutures on a twenty-first Dynasty mummy. Reproduced with permission from Majno G.[1]

rently, there are various types of absorbable and nonabsorbable sutures in different sizes with different-size needles; more than 40 different combinations are being used to close wounds and incisions.[3] Sutures provide a meticulous closure and have the greatest tensile

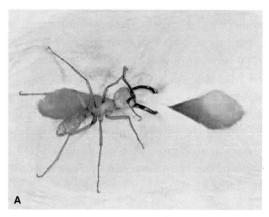
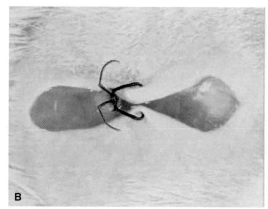

Majno G. The healing hand. Man and Wound in the Ancient World. 1975.

■ **FIGURE 1–2** *A* and *B*, Ant jaws closing a wound. Reproduced with permission from Majno G.[1]

strength and lowest dehiscence rate compared with any wound closure technique[4]; however, they are not without their disadvantages. The use of traumatic needles and the use of a foreign body to close a wound give them the highest infection rate as a wound closure device.[5,6] They also require the use of anesthesia and are a slow method of wound closure that is costly and difficult to master for some practitioners. In fact, many physicians and surgeons never acquire the ability to close wounds with sutures meticulously.[7] The use of needles can cause anxiety in patients and even in health care professionals, given the risk of transmitting bloodborne viruses such as human immunodeficiency virus (HIV) and hepatitis B and C.

Alternatives to sutures include staples, surgical tapes, and, most recently, tissue adhesives. Both staples and adhesive tapes have lower tissue reactivity than sutures and thus lower infection rates.[5,8] Staples are fast and have a low risk of a needle stick but require the use of anesthetics and, at times, can provide a less than meticulous cosmetic closure.[9] As with staples, adhesive tapes are fast and economical, in addition providing a painless closure that maximizes patient comfort; however, they have the lowest tensile strength and highest dehiscence rate of wound closure techniques, cannot be used inside the body around hair-bearing areas, and require the use of toxic adjuncts to maintain adherence to the skin.[10,11] Given the shortcomings of these wound closure devices, interest in tissue adhesives has grown in the last half-century and especially in the last decade. Tissue adhesives are now not only used as a method to close wounds but are being used to stop bleeding by sealing vascular structures, as topical wound sealants to provide an antimicrobial barrier to outside contamination, and to fixate structures where sutures and normal fixation devices such as plates and screws cannot be used.[12–16] The utility of tissue adhesives is so great that as this book is being written, countless more adhesives are being developed for use for numerous indications within the body.

CATEGORIES OF ADHESIVES AND DEFINITIONS

All products considered in this book are adhesives because, simply put, they stick. Different products vary in the mechanism and how well they stick, adhere, or bond. The specific mechanisms for each type of adhesive are described in each section. When evaluating how the adhesive sticks and how well it performs, it is important to clarify the terminology used to describe the adhesive, its mechanism, and its failure.

For the purpose of this book, we divided tissue adhesives into the categories of cyanoacrylate adhesives, fibrin-based adhesives, protein and synthetic polymers, and cements. These adhesives are distinct by their physical properties, so we have attributed separate chapters to each. The reader will also notice, however, that the indications for the various adhesives can overlap. For example, cyanoacrylate adhesives, fibrin-based adhesives, and protein polymers can all serve as sealants and as hemostatic agents. For that reason, it is important that we define the different uses of adhesives and their properties.

ADHESIVES AND SUBSTRATE

An adhesive is the material that does the sticking, and the material to which the adhesive bonds is called the substrate. For our purposes, this could be any tissue (skin, lung, liver, blood vessels).

TYPES OF BOND FAILURE

When the adhesive fails to bond the substrate together, the failure can be one of several modes. One is an adhesive failure, whereby the adhesive fails at the interface of the substrate. Another type of failure is a cohesive failure or material failure, whereby the adhesive fails within itself, and the third type of failure is a substrate failure, whereby the adhesive and cohesive bonds are so strong that the substrate or tissue fails. (Figure 1–3).

DEVICES, DRUGS, AND BIOLOGIC AGENTS: REGULATORY PATHWAYS AND LABELING

The US Food and Drug Administration (FDA) is mandated by the government to regulate all drugs and devices and is structured into several centers: one to handle devices, one to handle drugs, and another for biologic agents. Adhesives are generally considered devices and are handled by the section of the FDA dedicated to han-

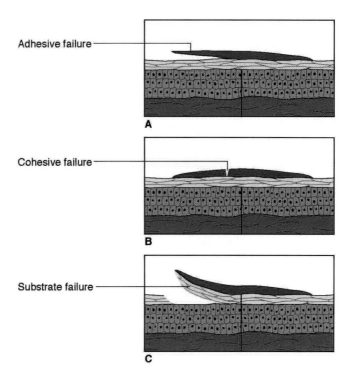

Adhesive failure

A

Cohesive failure

B

Substrate failure

C

■ **FIGURE 1-3** Types of bond failure.

dle devices, the Center for Devices and Radiologic Health (CDRH). Some adhesives with biologically active components (blood products), such as fibrin adhesives, are also regulated by the Center for Biologics Evaluation, and Research (CBER), which has expertise in blood, blood products, and cellular therapies, as well as the integral association of certain medical devices with these biologic products. Adhesives containing active drugs would be handled by the drug division of the FDA.

Devices are classified into three categories. Class I devices are subject to the least regulatory control. They present minimal potential for harm to the user and are often simpler in design than class II or III devices. The manufacturers of these products are subject to some general controls by the FDA (eg, they must provide evidence of good manufacturing practices), but exempt class I devices themselves are not regulated. Examples of class I exempt devices would be examination gloves and handheld surgical instruments. Class II devices are more complex devices. Some are exempt from premarket notification and control and have controls similar to those of class I devices that are considered nonexempt. Nonexempt class I and II devices need premarket notification, as do class III devices, which are the most stringent regulatory category for devices. Class III devices are those for which insufficient information exists to ensure safety and effectiveness solely through general or special controls. Class III devices are usually those that support or sustain human life, are of substantial importance in preventing impairment of human health, or present a potential, unreasonable risk of illness or injury.

Adhesives needing premarket approval (PMA) (class I and II nonexempt and class III) have two pathways to market in the United States. One is a full PMA, which is the FDA process of scientific and regulatory review to evaluate the safety and effectiveness of most class III medical devices. PMA is the most stringent type of device marketing application required by the FDA. The applicant must receive FDA approval of its PMA application prior to marketing the device. PMA is based on a determination by the FDA that the PMA contains sufficient valid scientific evidence to ensure that the device is safe and effective for its intended use(s). PMA is, in effect, a private license granting the applicant (or owner) permission to market the device. There are several phases to attaining PMA, including toxicologic studies, animal studies, and clinical trials that are approved and regulated by the FDA based on an investigational device exemption (IDE). Once these requirements are completed, FDA regulations provide 180 days to review the PMA and make a determination. In reality, the review time is normally longer. Before approving or denying a PMA, the appropriate FDA advisory committee may review the PMA at a public meeting and provide the FDA with the committee's recommendation on whether the FDA should approve the submission.

Another type of premarket notification or approval is the 510K. It comes from Section 510K of the Food, Drug and Cosmetic Act, which requires device manufacturers to notify the FDA, at least 90 days in advance, of their intent to market a medical device. It allows the FDA to determine whether the device is equivalent to a device already placed into one of the three classification categories. Thus, "new" devices (not in commercial distribution prior to May 28, 1976) that have not been classified can be properly identified. Specifically, medical device manufacturers are required to submit a premarket notification if they intend to introduce a device into commercial distribution for the first time or reintroduce a device that will be significantly changed or modified to the extent that its safety or effectiveness could be affected. Such change or modification could relate to the design, material, chemical composition, energy source, manufacturing process, or intended use.

We dedicated the final chapter in this book to a more comprehensive approach to the regulatory pathways of tissue adhesives from the FDA perspective.

CATEGORIES OF ADHESIVE USE

Hemostatic Agents

Anything that stops or impairs bleeding is a hemostatic agent. Thus, a hemostatic agent could be a mechanical agent (such as gauze or any surgical packing) or an adhesive acting as a sealant or embolic agent.[17,18] This can sometimes be confusing because sealants are often distinguished as a separate category to true tissue adhesives because they stick. Many of the sealants have low tensile strength and are used not as primary agents for wound closure but as adjuncts to anastomotic closure and to prevent flow or seepage of blood and body fluids.[14] However, stronger adhesives, such as cyanoacrylate adhesives, can also serve as sealants.[19] The reasons for the differentiation and semantics are multifactorial. One factor is the regulatory standards used and the goals of the manufacturer in the product claims.

Some also differentiate between hemostatics and adhesives based on the components in the device, not on the basis that they both stick. For example, fibrin sealants are often also called adhesives. They contain thrombin and fibrinogen, which, when combined, cross-link to form a sticky adhesive. This adhesive is relatively weak and is used primarily as a sealant and hemostatic agent but is also considered an adhesive. Other hemostatic agents will differentiate themselves from "fibrin adhesives" by containing only thrombin and depending on the fibrinogen from the patient's blood to cross-link and stick to their intended site, causing their hemostatic effect.

Sealants

Sealants are adhesives that prevent flow and seepage of blood or other body fluids. They can also be used to seal air leaks and have enjoyed more popularity with the advent of lung volume reduction

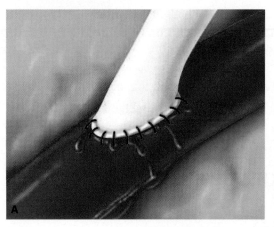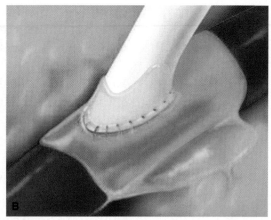

■ **Figure 1–4** *A* and *B*, Before and after use of sealants. Many different tissue adhesives can be used to seal vessels from leaking after anastomotic surgery.

surgery for emphysema.[20,21] By stopping the flow from leaking blood vessels, they can also be considered hemostatic agents. Several different adhesives from the categories discussed in this text can perform this function. Fibrin sealants and protein and synthetic polymers are both approved for this purpose.[13,14,22] To date, no cyanoacrylate adhesive is approved for this purpose by the FDA, but have been granted investigational device exemptions to begin clinical studies in this area (Figure 1–4).

Topical Wound Dressings

Adhesives applied as wound dressings for abrasions, burns, and surgical incisions are becoming more popular, and this popularity is likely to grow. Fibrin sealants have been studied and used extensively to help with burns and skin grafts, although they are not labeled or marketed for this purpose.[23–25] Cyanoacrylate adhesives are cheap and effective dressings. They seal wounds and burns, preventing further contamination, and reduce pain by sealing the wound.[26,27] Wound healing effectively occurs underneath the dressing of abrasions and burns treated with cyanoacrylate.[28–31] Numerous cyanoacrylate adhesives are now available to consumers as liquid bandages and as skin protectants.

Most wound dressings have been downgraded to class I devices. These dressings are nonexempt devices and need some premarket notification. The FDA had regulated wound dressing agents under regulation number 21 CFR §878.4490, "Absorbable Hemostatic Agents and Dressings." Although the name of the device classification includes "dressing," the FDA has interpreted this absorbable device as a surgical hemostatic agent. Wound dressings are topical, and some contain an indication for hemostasis and have been regulated as 510Ks for many years. The FDA recently modified the hemostatic classification to clarify that topical dressings are not included in the device classification of an absorbable hemostatic agent and are their own class of liquid bandages.

Wound Closure

The only adhesives approved for wound closure are the cyanoacrylate adhesives, which are approved only as topical wound closure devices.[6,32] An internal adhesive for wound closure that could act as an interface bond would have the potential for much better wound strength. However, issues such as allowing wound healing across a potential barrier would need to be addressed. To date, no implantable or absorbable adhesive has been approved for wound closure.

All cyanoacrylate adhesives approved for topical wound closure are considered class III transitional devices and require full PMA. Numerous studies have demonstrated the effectiveness and safety of cyanoacrylate adhesives for topical wound closure.[12,32,33] These devices may become declassified to class II devices when the FDA develops a level of comfort with these devices and the experience with their use for topical wound closure grows in the United States.

Embolic Agents

Adhesives have been used and approved as embolic agents.[34] Cyanocrylate adhesive is approved as a component of a device to embolize cerebral arteriovenous malformation as a class II device. There are also reports of cyanoacrylate adhesives being used to embolize gastric and esophageal varices, but these are off-label uses and are not approved by the FDA.[35-37] Care should be taken when considering the use of embolic agents in arteriovenous malformation because of the risk of pulmonary embolism.[38]

Fixation Devices

Cements have been used primarily as fixation devices to stabilize and fixate structures in the body, such as bones. Classic examples of these are the methacrylates used to fixate orthopedic prosthesis. Some cyanoacrylate adhesives are also considered cements and fixation devices, especially in the areas of dentistry and otolaryngology.[39-41]

Off-Label Uses Of Tissue Adhesives

Many uses for adhesives are described throughout this book. We have tried to describe reported uses and clearly document the FDA-approved uses and regulatory pathways for the various tissue adhesives and their indications. Occasionally, we refer to uses that have been reported but not approved by the FDA. In consideration of using a legally marketed device for a use other than how it is labeled, so-called "off-label use," a health care practitioner should be well informed about the product, use firm scientific rationale and sound medical evidence, and maintain records on the off-label use and its effects. The FDA is not responsible for regulating the practice of medicine and physicians. Thus, FDA approval is not needed for physicians to use any product; however, institutional review board approval may be necessary. Although many of the off-label uses described in the book may be safe, that safety is not ensured unless regulatory approval has been gained for the specific indication for which the product is intended to be used. Thus, none of the authors condone any off-label use of products mentioned in this book. Instead, we encourage practitioners to follow the regulatory guidance in Part 6 that outlines methods of gaining investigator approvals for specific situations that are not approved but in which they feel the use of adhesives may benefit their patients.

References

1. Majno G. The healing hand. Man and wound in the ancient world. Cambridge (MA): Harvard University Press; 1975.

2. Forrest RD. Early history of wound treatment. J R Soc Med 1982;75:198–205.

3. Wound closure manual. Somerville (NJ): Ethicon, Inc; 1985.

4. Cruse PJE, Ford R. A five-year prospective study of 23,649 surgical wounds. Arch Surg 1973;107:206–9.

5. Ritchie AJ, Rocke LG. Staples versus sutures in the closure of scalp wounds: a prospective, double-blind, randomized trial. Injury 1989;20:217–8.

6. Quinn JV, Maw JL, Ramotar K, et al. Octylcyanoacrylate tissue adhesive wound repair versus suture wound repair in a contaminated wound model. Surgery 1997;122:69–72.

7. Singer AJ, Hollander JE, Valentine SM, et al. Association of training level and short-term cosmetic appearance of repaired lacerations.

Acad Emerg Med 1996;3:378–83.

8. Johnson A, Rodeheaver GT, Durand LS, et al. Automatic disposable stapling devices for wound closure. Ann Emerg Med 1981;10:631–5.

9. George TK, Simpson DC. Skin wound closure with staples in the accident and emergency department. J R Coll Surg Edinb 1985;30:54–6.

10. Rothnie NG, Taylor GW. Suture less skin closure. A clinical trial. BMJ 1963;5364:1027–30.

11. Panek PH, Prusak MP, Bolt D, Edlich RF. Potentiation of wound infection by adhesive adjuncts. Am Surg 1972;38:343–5.

12. Quinn JV, Wells GA, Sutcliffe T, et al. A randomized trial comparing octylcyanoacrylate tissue adhesive and sutures in the management of lacerations. JAMA 1997;277:1527–30.

13. Chao HH, Torchiana DF. BioGlue: albumin/glutaraldehyde sealant in cardiac surgery. J Card Surg 2003;18:500–3.

14. Glickman M, Gheissari A, Money S, et al. A polymeric sealant inhibits anastomotic suture hole bleeding more rapidly than Gelfoam/thrombin: results of a randomized controlled trial. Arch Surg 2002; 137:326–31.

15. Tock B, Drohan W, Hess J, et al. Haemophilia and advanced fibrin sealant technologies. Haemophilia 1998;4:449–55.

16. Jackson M, MacPhee M, Drohan W, Alving B. Fibrin sealant: current and potential clinical applications. Blood Coagul Fibrinolysis 1996;7:737–46.

17. Jackson MR, Friedman SA, Carter AJ, et al. Hemostatic efficacy of a fibrin sealant-based topical agent in a femoral artery injury model: a randomized, blinded, placebo-controlled study. J Vasc Surg 1997; 26:274–80.

18. Holcomb J, Pusateri A, Hess J, et al. Implications of new dry fibrin sealant technology for trauma surgery. Surg Clin North Am 1997; 77:943–52.

19. Collins JA, James PM, Levitsky SA, et al. Cyanoacrylate adhesives as topical hemostatic aids. II. Clinical use in seven combat casualties. Surgery 1969;65:260–3.

20. Glover W, Chavis TV, Daniel TM, et al. Fibrin glue application through the flexible fiberoptic bronchoscope: closure of bronchopleural fistulas. J Thorac Cardiovasc Surg 1987;93:470–2.

21. Keller CA. Lasers, staples, bovine pericardium, talc, glue and…suction cylinders? Tools of the trade to avoid air leaks in lung volume reduction surgery. Chest 2004;125:361–3.

22. Milne AA, Murphy WG, Reading SJ, Ruckley CV. Fibrin sealant reduces suture line bleeding during carotid endarterectomy: a randomised trial. Eur J Vasc Endovasc Surg 1995;10:91–4.

23. Saltz R, Sierra D, Feldman D, et al. Experimental and clinical applica-

tions of fibrin glue. Plast Reconstr Surg 1991;88:1005–15; discussion 1016–7.

24. Saltz R, Dimick A, Harris C, et al. Application of autologous fibrin glue in burn wounds. J Burn Care Rehabil 1989;10:504–7.

25. Saltz R, Zamora S. Tissue adhesives and applications in plastic and reconstructive surgery. Aesthetic Plast Surg 1998;22:439–43.

26. Singer A, Berrutti L, Thode HJ, McClain S. Octylcyanoacrylate for the treatment of partial-thickness burns in swine: a randomized, controlled experiment. Acad Emerg Med 1999;6:688–92.

27. Singer AJ, Mohammad M, Tortora G, et al. Octylcyanoacrylate for the treatment of contaminated partial-thickness burns in swine: a randomized controlled experiment. Acad Emerg Med 2000;7:222–7.

28. Quinn J, Lowe L, Mertz M. The effect of a new tissue-adhesive wound dressing on the healing of traumatic abrasions. Dermatology 2000;201:343–6.

29. Singer A, Berrutti L, McClain S. Comparative trial of octyl-cyanoacrylate and silver sulfadiazine for the treatment of full-thickness skin wounds. Wound Repair Regen 1999;7:356–61.

30. Singer AJ, Nable M, Cameau P, et al. Evaluation of a new liquid occlusive dressing for excisional wounds. Wound Repair Regen 2003;11:181–7.

31. Singer A, Thode H Jr, McClain S. The effects of octylcyanoacrylate on scarring after burns. Acad Emerg Med 2001;8:107–11.

32. Quinn JV, Drzewiecki A, Li MM, et al. A randomized, controlled trial comparing a tissue adhesive with suturing in the repair of pediatric facial lacerations. Ann Emerg Med 1993;22:1130–5.

33. Singer AJ, Hollander JE, Valentine SM, et al. Prospective randomized controlled trial of a new tissue adhesive (2-octylcyanoacrylate) versus standard wound closure techniques for laceration repair. Acad Emerg Med 1998;5:94–8.

34. n-Butyl cyanoacrylate embolization of cerebral arteriovenous malformations: results of a prospective, randomized, multi-center trial. AJNR Am J Neuroradiol 2002;23:748–55.

35. Lunderquist A, Borjesson B, Owman T, Bengmark S. Isobutyl 2-cyanoacrylate (bucrylate) in obliteration of gastric coronary vein and esophageal varices. AJR Am J Roentgenol 1978;130:1–6.

36. Mostafa I, Omar MM, Nouh A. Endoscopic control of gastric variceal bleeding with butyl cyanoacrylate in patients with schistosomiasis. J Egypt Soc Parasitol 1997;27:405–10.

37. Arakaki Y, Murakami K, Takahashi K, et al. Clinical evaluation of combined endoscopic variceal ligation and sclerotherapy of gastric varices in liver cirrhosis. Endoscopy 2003;35:940–5.

38. Carapiet DA, Stevens JE. Pulmonary embolism following embolization of an arteriovenous malformation. Paediatr Anaesth 1996;6:491–4.

39. Siedentop K. Reconstruction of ossicles by tissue glue histoacryl in dogs. Laryngoscope 1974;84:1397–403.

40. Maw JL, Kartush JM. Ossicular chain reconstruction using a new tissue adhesive. Am J Otol 2000;21:301–5.

41. Maw JL, Kartush JM, Bouchard K, Raphael Y. Octylcyanoacrylate: a new medical-grade adhesive for otologic surgery. Am J Otol 2000;21:310–4.

2 History and Background

GEORGE J. MATTAMAL, PHD

Currently, tissue adhesives and glues are an alternative technology in clinical applications that are important both to the medical industry and the surgical profession. Many of these emerging tissue adhesives can modify difficult surgical procedures by stabilizing tissue surfaces through hemostasis, sealing of wounds, and fixation of tissue in areas inaccessible to staples, clips, and suture placement. Currently, physicians have relied heavily on sutures, clips, and staples, which have an estimated annual worldwide market of over $2.5 billion for wound closure alone.[1] There have been significant advances in this technology because of excellent clinical research and development in this field during the last 15 years.

In a broad sense, tissue adhesives and glues can be categorized into biologic, composite (hybrid) biologic, synthetic, and genetically engineered polymer protein glues. A biologic tissue adhesive is a natural substance consisting of blood products, for example, Fibrin Sealant (Tisseel VH Kit).* It is used as "an adjunct to hemostasis in surgeries involving cardiopulmonary bypass and treatment of splenic injuries due to blunt or penetrating trauma to the abdomen, when control of bleeding by conventional surgical techniques, including suture, ligature, and cautery, is ineffective or impractical; [it is] also indicated as an adjunct for the closure of colostomies…"* Tisseel is manufactured using fibrinogen as the main ingredient (a protein from human blood that forms a clot), thrombin (another blood protein that facilitates

*Fibrin Sealant (Tisseel VH Kit), manufactured by Oesterreichisches Institut Fuer Haemoderivate G.M.B.H. in Vienna, Austria, and distributed by Baxter Healthcare Corporation, Glendale, CA, was approved [Biologics License 2.55 in accordance with the provisions of Section 351(a) of the Public Health Service Act] by the US Food and Drug Administration (FDA) on May 1, 1998.

blood clotting), bovine fibrinolysis inhibitor solution, and other clotting factors or additives. An example of a composite (hybrid) biologic tissue adhesive is BioGlue Surgical Adhesive.[†] It is a two-component (natural and synthetic substance) system consisting of purified bovine serum albumin and glutaraldehyde. It is indicated for use "as an adjunct to standard methods of achieving hemostasis (such as sutures and staples) in adult patients in open surgical repair of large vessels (such as aorta, femoral, and carotid arteries)."[†] Synthetic tissue adhesives and glues include cyanoacrylate tissue adhesives, such as Dermabond (Closure Medical Corporation, Raleigh, NC), Indermil Tissue Adhesive (United States Surgical, a Division of Tyco Healthcare Group, L.P., Norwalk, CT), and Histoacryl Blue (B. Braun, Melsungen AG, Melsungen, Germany),[‡] and polymeric sealants, such as FocalSeal-L Synthetic Absorbable Sealant[§] and CoSeal Surgical Sealant.[||] Genetically engineered polymer protein glues are polymers that are based on protein engineering and deoxyribonucleic acid (DNA) gene technology, which are still at experimental stages.

PHYSICAL AND CHEMICAL PROPERTIES OF SYNTHETIC CYANOACRYLATE ADHESIVES

Synthetic cyanocrylate adhesives (alkyl-2-cyanoacrylates or alkyl-α-cyanoacrylates) are a family of liquid monomers[2] consisting of the alkyl esters of 2-cyanoacrylic acid. They polymerize at room temperature in an exothermic reaction, releasing heat in the process, on contact with a small amount of water or basic fluid to form polymers, poly(alkyl-2-cyanoacrylates). They form strong adhesive bonds with a variety of substrates, such as wood, metal, hard tissue (ie, bone and enamel), and soft tissue (ie, skin, vascular tissue).

[†]BioGlue Surgical Adhesive (P010003), manufactured by Cryolife, Inc., Kennesaw, GA, was approved on October 8, 2002.
[‡]Histoacryl Blue has been sold widely since 1980 in Canada and Europe only.
[§]FocalSeal-L Synthetic Absorbable Sealant (P990028) was approved on May 26, 2000. It is based on polyethylene glycol (PEG) hydrogel technology. It is composed of a synthetic absorbable sealant and primer aqueous solutions of PEG that have been modified with short segments of acrylate-capped poly(L-lactide) and poly(trimethylene carbonate). It is intended for use as an adjunct to standard closure of visceral pleural air leaks incurred during elective pulmonary resection.
[||]CoSeal Surgical Sealant (P010022) was approved on December 14, 2001. It is based on polyethylene glycol (PEG) hydrogel technology. It is formed when two synthetic derivatized PEG polymers are mixed together and applied to tissue. It is designed to act as a vascular sealant and is indicated for use in vascular reconstructions to achieve adjunctive hemostasis by mechanically sealing areas of leakage.

Different synthetic cyanoacrylate adhesives (alkyl-2-cyanoacrylates) can be manufactured by altering the alkoxycarbonyl group (–COOR) of the molecule. Most methods involve a condensation of formaldehyde ($H_2C=O$) with an alkyl cyanoacetate ($N\equiv C–CH_2–COOR$) in the presence of a base catalyst (such as piperidine) to form a low-molecular-weight cyanoacrylic ester polymer, poly(alkyl-2-cyanoacrylate). This polymer is then depolymerized (cracked) in the presence of a polymerization inhibitor (such as phosphorous pentoxide, nitric oxide, sulfur dioxide) at a high temperature by heating to distill off the liquid cyanoacrylate adhesive monomer alkyl-2-cyanoacrylate. It is further purified by several consecutive fractional distillations, eliminating reactants and any unused materials that may cause premature polymerization. The liquid cyanoacrylate monomer is then stabilized with a free radical inhibitor, such as hydroquinone, which is a free radical trap preventing repolymerization. Finally, various cyanoacrylate adhesive formulations can be manufactured by varying viscosity, spreadability, set time, bond strength, degradation rate, and other physical, chemical, and mechanical properties of the cyanaoacrylate monomers. Over 90% of cyanoacrylate adhesive formulations will be of the pure liquid monomer alkyl-2-cyanoacrylate. The other formulation components are added to obtain appropriate performance of the desired final products. They include stabilizers (to prolong the shelf life of the formation), polymerization inhibitors (to delay the transition from liquid formulation to solid polymer), and plasticizers (to maximize the strength and flexibility of the polymer after application, such as in the case of topical skin application products).

CHEMICAL STRUCTURES OF CYANOACRYLATE MONOMERS

Synthetic cyanoacrylate monomers have been available since 1951; however, their clinical use has been limited because of the potential for thermal damage and scarring to the tissues by heat generation (exothermic reaction) as they transform from monomeric to polymeric form and concerns about the cytotoxic or histotoxic effects of the by-products resulting from the degradation of polymer, poly(alkyl-2-cyanoacrylate), which include, notably, formaldehyde and the corresponding alkyl cyanoacetate and other breakdown products.

Although the polymerized cyanoacrylate monomer[3] gains adhesion rather quickly, the curing process results in tight bonds being formed, and some polymers can lack flexibility. Electronegative groups such as the nitrile ($-C\equiv N$) and alkoxycarbonyl ($-COOR$) groups of the alkyl-2-cyanoacrylate monomer make the monomer extremely reactive (Figure 2–1). These groups enhance anionic polymerization at ambient temperatures even with very weak bases, such as water.

The alkyl side chain ($-R$) determines the rate of degradation, rate of polymerization with release of heat in the process, toxicity, flexibility, and the properties of the adhesive formed when a monomer polymerizes into a polymer. For example, earlier clinical studies revealed that when the side chain ($-R$) of the cyanoacrylate monomers was short, such as in methyl-2-cyanoacrylate, it polymerized quickly to give a rigid polymer matrix, poly(methyl-2-cyanoacrylate), and degraded rapidly into corresponding alkyl cyanoacetate and formaldehyde, which can lead to significant histotoxicity.[4,5] The degradation of the polymer also depends on the molecular weight of the polymer formed; a lower-molecular-weight polymer, poly(methyl-2-cyanoacrylate), degrades more rapidly into corresponding alkyl cyanoacetate, formaldehyde, and other breakdown products. On the other hand, when cyanoacrylate monomers with longer alkyl chains (ie, higher homologues), such as n-butyl-2-cyanoacrylate and 2-octyl-cyanoacrylate, polymerize slowly, they form flexible polymers and degrade slowly to form fewer toxic degradation products. Accordingly, longer-chain cyanoacrylate monomers are considered to be less toxic owing to their slower degradation when compared with their shorter side chain counterparts. The formation of toxic degraded products of the polymer poly(alkyl-2-cyanoacrylate) decreases with an increase in the length of the alkyl side chain ($-R$) and molecular weight of the polymer.

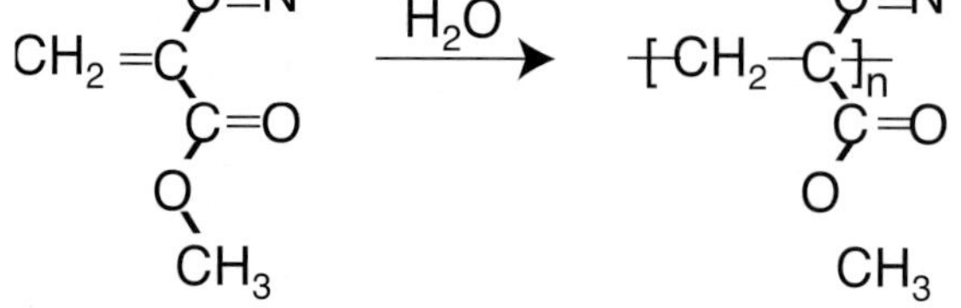

■ FIGURE 2–1 Chemical structures of cyanoacrylate monomers.

Coover discovered the adhesive properties of synthetic cyanoacrylates (alkyl-2-cyanoacrylates) in the research laboratories of the Tennessee Eastman Company in 1951.[6] Several years later, in 1958, this discovery led Eastman Kodak to the introduction of the first cyanoacrylate adhesive, methyl-2-cyanoacrylate, called Eastman 910 Adhesive, into the commercial market. In the meantime, Coover did extensive research to develop tissue adhesives based on cyanoacrylate homologues through collaboration with Ethicon Company (Somerville, NJ). Coover applied for US Food and Drug Administration (FDA) approval for one of the cyanoacrylate monomers as a tissue adhesive in 1964.[2] He was, however, unable to obtain FDA approval, and, in 1970, he discontinued his work in medical applications of cyanoacrylate tissue adhesives. At the same time, alkyl-2-cyanoacrylates, such as n-butyl-2-cyanoacrylate monomer, were made in Europe, Japan, Israel, and Canada. Many clinical experiences on the use of n-butyl-2-cyanoacrylate, such as Histoacryl Blue, were reported, namely, for its clinical use in wound closure, such as for traumatic lacerations and surgical incisions (Table 2–1). Accordingly, Histoacryl Blue was the first cyanoacrylate tissue adhesive used clinically for closure of skin incisions in Europe and Canada in the early 1980s.[4]

In the United States, since 1998, the FDA has approved the following three class III premarket approval (PMA) devices associated with cyanoacrylate monomers (see Chapter 8, "US Food and Drug Administration Perspective on Class I, II, and III Cyanoacrylate Medical Devices"):

1. On August 26, 1998, the FDA approved the first class III tissue adhesive device for topical skin approximation, Dermabond (P960052). It is composed of over 90% 2-octyl-cyanoacrylate monomer, the balance being a plasticizer, a radical stabilizer, an

Table 2–1 Various Cyanoacrylate Adhesive Products

R	Name	Trade Name
$-CH_3$	Methyl-2-cyanoacrylate	Eastman 910 Adhesive
$-C_2H_5$	Ethyl-2-cyanoacrylate	Krazy Glue
$-C_4H_9$	n-Butyl-2-cyanoacrylate	Indermil Tissue Adhesive Trufill Liquid Embolic Agent Histoacryl Blue*
$-C_8H_{17}$	2-Octyl-cyanoacrylate	Dermabond

*Sold widely since 1980 in Canada and Europe only.

anionic stabilizer, and colorant. Polymerized Dermabond will slough off from the skin as the wound reepithelializes, usually within 5 to 10 days. The intended use of Dermabond is for "topical application to hold closed easily approximated skin edges from surgical incisions, including punctures from minimally invasive surgery, and simple, thoroughly cleaned, trauma-induced lacerations. Dermabond may be used in conjunction with, but not in place of, subcuticular sutures." Closure Medical Corporation conducted a prospective, randomized, controlled, and unmasked clinical trial involving 769 patients.[7] The study was conducted to evaluate the safety and effectiveness of closing approximated skin edges of surgical incisions, including punctures from minimally invasive surgery, and trauma-induced lacerations using Dermabond in comparison with US Pharmacopeia (USP) size 5 to 0 or smaller suture, adhesive strips, or staples, with or without dermal closure (subcuticular suture), as per the clinical investigator's judgment. The outcome of these clinical studies, along with other physical and mechanical tests and preclinical studies, including laboratory animal tests (adhesion and tensile strength), was reviewed by the Center for Devices and Radiological Health (CDRH) (see Chapter 7, "US Food and Drug Administration Perspective on the Regulation of Medical Device Tissue Adhesives," and Chapter 8, "US Food and Drug Administration Perspective on Class I, II, and III Cyanoacrylate Medical Devices"), one of the six centers within the FDA, and presented to the General and Plastic Surgery Devices Panel for review and recommendation on January 30, 1998. The panel determined that the data provide reasonable assurance that the class III tissue adhesive device Dermabond is safe and effective when used in accordance with the labeling. The FDA approved Dermabond for commercial distribution on August 26, 1998.

2. On May 22, 2002, the FDA approved the second cyanoacrylate tissue adhesive for topical skin approximation, Indermil Tissue Adhesive (P010002). It is composed of over 90% n-butyl-2-cyanoacrylate monomer, the balance being a plasticizer, a radical stabilizer, and an anionic stabilizer. Polymerized Indermil Tissue Adhesive, a cyanoacrylate monomer that is similar to Dermabond, will slough off from the skin as the wound reepithelializes, usually within 5 to 10 days. The intended use of Indermil Tissue Adhesive is "for closure of topical skin incisions including laparoscopic incisions, and trauma-induced lacerations in areas of low skin tension that are simple, thoroughly-cleansed, and have easily approximated skin edges. Indermil may be used in conjunction with, but not in place of, deep dermal stitches."

United States Surgical conducted a multicenter, prospective, randomized clinical trial involving 24 sites and 1,092 patients. This randomized trial compared Indermil Tissue Adhesive with traditional wound closure techniques (sutures, staples, and adhesive strips) to evaluate the safety and effectiveness of wound closure of patients with surgical incisions or lacerations of 8 cm or less that were treated and assessed for complication (dehiscence, infection, skin irritation), time to wound closure, and cosmesis (the cosmetic appearance of the wound after 3 months). The outcome of the clinical studies, along with other physical and mechanical tests and preclinical studies, including laboratory animal tests, was reviewed by the CDRH (see Chapters 7 and 8). Pursuant to section 515(c) (2) of the Food and Cosmetic Act, as amended by the Safe Medical Devices Act of 1990, this PMA was not referred to the General and Plastic Surgery Devices Panel. The rationale for this was that the FDA had determined that this PMA substantially duplicated information previously reviewed by this panel for Dermabond (P960052). On May 22, 2002, the CDRH determined that the data provide reasonable assurance that the class III tissue adhesive device Indermil Tissue Adhesive is safe and effective when used in accordance with the labeling, and the FDA approved Indermil Tissue Adhesive for commercial distribution.

3. On September 25, 2000, the FDA approved the first class III cyanoacrylate monomer for neurologic embolization (P990040), Trufill n-Butyl Cyanoacrylate (n-BCA) Liquid Embolic System (Cordis Neurovascular, Inc., Miami Lakes, FL). It is formulated of n-butyl-2-cyanoacrylate monomer (over 90% with other ingredients), ethiodized oil, and tantalum powder. It is a three-component system that is not intended to be used separately. Specifically, the composition of the three-component embolic agent is a mixture of tantalum power and ethiodized oil, which are mixed with n-butyl-2-cyanoacrylate monomer (n-BCA). The principle behind the device's operation is to block the supply of blood to a vascular lesion so that the lesion may be surgically removed with increased safety to the patient. This mixture is placed in cerebral arteriovenous malformations (AVMs) via an arterial catheter using fluoroscopy. Specifically, it is used under fluoroscopic guidance to obstruct or reduce the blood flow to AVMs via superselective catheter delivery. On contact with body fluids or tissue, the three-component mixture polymerizes into a solid material. Ethiodized oil (an oily fluid containing iodinated poppy seed oil) is a radiopaque polymerizing retardant and will vary the rate of polymerization of n-BCA. The finely ground dark gray

metal tantalum powder is used to provide additional radiopacification to the n-BCA and ethiodized oil mixture. Specifically, n-BCA is intended to occlude AVMs, whereas tantalum powder and ethiodized oil are intended to opacify this vascular lesion. The intended use of the Trufill n-Butyl Cyanoacrylate (n-BCA) Liquid Embolic System is for "the embolization of cerebral [AVMs] when presurgical devasculation is desired." The safety and effectiveness of this embolic system class III device as a long-term implant have not been established. The three-component mixture (n-BCA + ethiodized oil + tantalum powder) that was polymerized was not intended to be left in the brain because the purpose of the device is to preoperatively prepare the AVM for surgical removal of both the embolic agent and the AVM. Accordingly, as recommended by the Neurological Devices Advisory Panel, the labeling of this device contains a warning regarding long-term implantation, such as "not intended to be a permanent implant in the body."

Cordis Neurovascular, Inc. conducted a prospective, randomized, single-blind clinical trial involving 104 patients at 13 sites. The study was conducted to evaluate if the Trufill n-Butyl Cyanoacrylate (n-BCA) Liquid Embolic System was as safe and effective as the control device, polyvinyl alcohol particles (Trufill PVA), for use in the obliteration of cerebral AVMs when presurgical devascularization was desired. The outcome of this clinical study, along with other physical and mechanical tests and preclinical studies, including laboratory animal tests, was reviewed by the CDRH (see Chapters 7 and 8) and on May 11, 2000, was presented to the Neurological Devices Advisory Panel for review and recommendation. The panel determined that the data provide reasonable assurance that the class III device Trufill n-Butyl Cyanoacrylate (n-BCA) Liquid Embolic System is safe and effective when used in accordance with the labeling of this device that incorporates a warning regarding long-term implantation, such as "not intended to be a permanent implant in the body." The FDA approved the Trufill n-Butyl Cyanoacrylate (n-BCA) Liquid Embolic System on September 25, 2000, for commercial distribution.

FDA RECOMMENDATIONS FOR TESTING OF CYANOACRYLATE TISSUE ADHESIVE FOR TOPICAL APPROXIMATION OF SKIN

On February 13, 2004, the FDA published a guidance document entitled "Guidance for Industry and FDA Staff, Cyanoacrylate Tissue Adhesive for Topical Approximation of Skin – Premarket Approval Applications (PMAs)."[8] The FDA developed this guidance document based on its review experience, published scientific clinical articles, and input from the General and Plastic Surgery Advisory Panel and manufacturers of these types of devices. The document provides guidance to regulatory personnel and manufacturers in the preparation of investigational device exemption (IDE) applications and in the development of valid scientific evidence to support PMA applications for cyanoacrylate topical tissue adhesives. Specifically, this guidance document identifies important preclinical, clinical, and labeling information that should be submitted in marketing applications (ie, PMAs or product development protocol).[9]

The cyanoacrylate guidance document is intended to provide useful information for helping manufacturers to meet FDA regulatory requirements. The manufacturers may consider factors such as final product release specifications, which include viscosity determination; analysis of the residual content of the components of bulk formation by gas chromatography, nuclear magnetic resonance, and mass spectrometry; determination of residual levels of manufacturing reagents; purity of the final product; moisture determination; setting time determination; heat of polymerization determination; physical, chemical, and mechanical testing; sterility testing; and stability or shelf life determination. Polymerization of liquid cyanoacrylate tissue adhesives is an exothermic reaction, and the temperature rise in surrounding tissue is governed by the rate of curing (polymerization) and thickness of the adhesive material applied to the surgical site. Viscosity, setting time, and adhesive performance of cyanoacrylate liquid monomers are major factors that define the utility of the final product. The viscosity of the liquid adhesive in the final product is a primary indicator of the stability of the final product. As cyanoacrylate adhesive formation ages, the viscosity increases owing to the transition of the monomer into polymer (see Figure 2–1). This, in effect, reduces the concentration of monomer and can affect the adhesive bond formed with the underlying tissue. Thus, key adhesive properties, such as tensile strength, tensile or overlap shear strength, peel adhesion strength, and impact strength, may be evaluated by performing appropriate tests on the final cyanoacrylate adhesive product. Setting time is influenced by the stability of the final product and is the basis for specific instructions for the physician applying the product.

Aside from the general biocompatibility testing, this guidance document recommends additional animal testing of cyanoacrylate topical tissue adhesives, such as the animal studies to evaluate the potential for delayed healing using histopathology. The FDA recommends that animal tests represent the method of applications that will be used in human studies and that the amount of the product used in the animal study be compared with that proposed for use in humans. The FDA considers that cyanoacrylate topical tissue adhesives are "significant risk devices" and that clinical studies of the same must be conducted under IDE regulation 21 CFR Part 812 (see Chapters 7 and 8). The FDA recommends a feasibility study (a small, usually nonrandomized, one- or two-site study), which may be used to evaluate the procedures to be used in the pivotal study, that is, refine instructions for use, and/or provide initial experience to potential investigators. The data derived from a feasibility study are critical toward meeting FDA regulatory recommendations in the design of the pivotal trial toward estimating the treatment effect and establishing the appropriate sample size for the pivotal safety and effectiveness study.

OTHER USE OF CYANOACRYLATE ADHESIVES

A recent search of the literature revealed several references to various uses of cyanoacrylate adhesives, many of which have not been approved and/or cleared by the FDA. For example, this includes hundreds of *Cambridge Scientific Abstracts* over the last 17 years, 295 scientific abstracts from *TOXNET* from 1966 to the present, 1,638 citations from *Science Direct*, 59 abstracts from *INSPEC* from 1969 to the present, 18 articles from *Health Devices Alerts Abstract*, and numerous other published clinical articles over a period of 30 years. These sources reveal that synthetic cyanoacrylate tissue adhesives have been used extensively as an alternative to current conventional treatments in clinical applications and studies, including applications in thoracic, gastrointestinal, neurologic, cardiovascular, ophthalmologic, and vascular surgery. They also include the use of cyanoacrylates for embolization in neurologic, urologic, and cardiovascular procedures and for cartilage and bone grafting procedures. For example, it was reported in the standard treatments of AVM that the strong adhesive force of cyanoacrylate derivatives sometimes glues the tip of the microcatheter to the artery, resulting in serious complications[10]; moreover, the organic solvents used to dissolve polymers cause damage to the surrounding brain tissue of an AVM. It has also been reported that implantation of cyanoacrylate tissue adhesive into subcutaneous tissues can result in an acute inflammatory response and foreign-body giant cell reaction.[11] Cyanoacrylates have been reported to have variable toxicity when implanted and used for procedures such as nerve and cartilage grafts. This toxicity appears to be more apparent in vascular areas but is also largely due to the cyanoacrylate formulation used.

Cyanoacrylate properties vary greatly, depending on the formulation. Therefore, before various cyanoacrylate monomers can be used successfully, their properties and the potential adverse events of each different cyanoacrylate tissue adhesive formulation must be characterized before they may be used for permanent implantation in patients. As explained in this chapter, currently, the FDA has approved the Trufill Embolic System for aiding neurologic embolization. The safety and effectiveness of the Trufill Embolic System device as a long-term implant have not been established. Hence, there are no current cyanoacrylate tissue adhesives approved in the United States by the FDA for long-term implantation in the human body. To design new biodegradable or bioabsorbable cyanoacrylate tissue adhesives, issues must be addressed that are pertinent to their flexibility, setting time, bond strength, heat of polymerization, viscosity, toxicity, biocompatibility, sterility, biodegradable or bioabsorbable profile, and stability or shelf life. However, animal studies have shown promise in revealing that the cyanoacrylate adhesives degrade gradually in vivo and are eliminated naturally by excretion, leaving no measurable levels of toxic breakdown products in the surrounding healthy tissues.[12–15] These types of animal studies eventually will provide insights into the design of future biodegradable or bioabsorbable cyanoacrylate tissue adhesives that may have the potential to be implanted into the human body for clinical applications.

In summary, the long-term effects of cyanoacrylate tissue adhesives for permanent implantation in the tissues, such as vascularized tissue, are presently unknown. In the future, preclinical and clinical studies may ultimately shed more light on the suitability of the cyanoacrylate monomers for permanent implantation in the human body.

REFERENCES

1. Webster AIN, Peter J. Adhesives for medical applications. In: Dumitriu S, editor. Polymeric biomaterials. 2nd ed rev. New York: Marcel Dekker, Inc; 2002. p. 703–37.

2. Chu CC, von Fraunhofer JA, Greisler HP. Wound closure biomaterials and devices. New York: CRC Press, Inc.; 1997.

3. Matsumoto T. Tissue adhesives in surgery. New York: Medical Examination Publishing Co., Inc.; 1972.

4. Quinn JV. Tissue adhesives in wound care. Hamilton (ON): BC Decker Inc; 1998.

5. Trott A. Cyanoacrylate tissue adhesives [editorial]. JAMA 1997; 277:1559–60.

6. Coover. HW Jr, Joyner FB, Shearer NH, Wicker TH. Chemistry and performance of cyanoacrylate adhesives. Soc Plast Eng J 1959;15:413–7.

7. Singer AJ, Quinn JV, Hollander JE. Comparison of octylcyanoacrylate and standard wound closure methods for lacerations and incisions. Surgery 2002;131:270–6.

8. US Food and Drug Administration. Guidance for industry and FDA staff, cyanoacrylate tissue adhesive for topical approximation of skin – premarket approval applications (PMAs), February 13, 2004. Available at: http://www.fda.gov/cdrh/ode/guidance/1233.html (accessed Feb 13, 2004).

9. US Food and Drug Administration. Guidance for industry, contents of a product development protocol, July 27, 1998. Available at: www.fda.gov/cdrh/pdp/pdpguide.pdf (accessed July 27, 1998).

10. Kazekawa K, Iwata H, Shimozuru T, et al. Nontoxic embolic liquids for treatment of arteriovenous malformations. J Biomed Mater Res 1997;38:79–86.

11. Forseth M, O' Grady K, Toriumi DM. Current status of cyanoacrylate and fibrin tissue adhesives. J Long Term EFF Med Implant 1992;2:221–33.

12. Kulkarni RK, Hanks GA, Pani KC, Leonard F. The in vivo metabolic degradation of poly (methyl cyanoacrylate) via thiocyanate. J Biomed Mater Res 1967;1:11–6.

13. Pani KC, Gladieux G, Brandes G, et al. The degradation of n-butyl alpha-cyanoacrylate tissue adhesive. II. Surgery 1968;63:481–9.

14. Wade CW, Leonard F. Degradation of poly (methyl 2-cyanoacrylates). J Biomed Mater Res 1972;6:215–20.

15. Cameron JL, Woodward SC, Pulaski EJ, et al. The degradation of cyanoacrylate tissue adhesive. Surgery 1965;58:424.

3 Clinical Approaches to the Use of Cyanoacrylate Tissue Adhesives

James V. Quinn, MD, MS

Cyanoacrylate adhesives were first synthesized in 1949.[1] They have tremendous tensile strength and have enjoyed great success as commercial "superglues."

In the 1950s and 1960s, cyanoacrylate adhesives were used to close wounds and bond other human tissue. When implanted, it was evident that the short-chain monomers used were histotoxic, demonstrating acute and chronic inflammatory reactions primarily as the result of foreign-body reactions.[2] These foreign-body reactions have been noted to be greater when the implantation of material was in an area of high vascularity.[3] It was found that rapidly polymerizing and degrading short-chain monomers caused histotoxicity secondary to the heat of polymerization and the high concentration of breakdown products.

Over time, it was determined that long-chain polymers could be used topically to hold wounds together without any significant toxicity.[4] Degradation was slower with the long-chain monomers, and they sloughed off before any significant degradation or toxicity occurred. However, much about cyanoacrylate adhesives remained a mystery; their medical applications were poorly studied, and the Food and Drug Administration (FDA) in the United States was slow and hesitant to approve these substances. During the 1970s and 1980s, they became popular choices for treating wounds in Europe, Israel, the Far East, and Canada.[5–7] In these countries, they demonstrated a history of safety for more than 25 years before the FDA approved the first product for topical use in 1998 and a second product in 2002.

With the recent approvals by the FDA, manufacturers of medical devices now have the incentive to innovate cyanoacrylate formulations, applicators, and application techniques to optimize the medical applications for these adhesives. As a result, numerous other formulations have been approved or are pending approval from the FDA for numerous indications.

CHEMICAL STRUCTURE AND PHYSICAL PROPERTIES

Over the last few years, more and more cyanoacrylate products have become available to health care professionals, and this number will continue to increase over the next few years. To select and properly use the right cyanoacrylate adhesive for the appropriate clinical situation, it is important to understand how the different formulations work and how their properties separate them from other formulations and make them optimal for a particular indication. Although all cyanoacrylates arise from the same basic structure, subtle variations can dramatically change the properties of the compounds.[2,8] By incorporating other materials, such as viscosifying agents, plasticizers, and initiators, the indications and contraindications for each monomer and formulation can vary tremendously with small changes in the chemical structure or additions to the formulation.

CHEMISTRY OF THE MONOMER

The basic chemical structure is consistent for the family of cyanoacrylate adhesives, but the alkyl or carbon side chain has an important impact on the properties and eventual performance of the adhesive (Figure 3–1).

In general, the shorter the alkyl side chain, the more branches off the side chain, or the more oxygen molecules incorporated into the alkyl chain (eg, methyl, ethyl, methoxyl), the more reactive the compound. A highly reactive compound will set fast and be extremely strong. However, this strength does not always equate to a stronger bond because short-chain monomers tend to form tight, brittle bonds, which can fracture easily. Also, short-chain monomers, when exposed

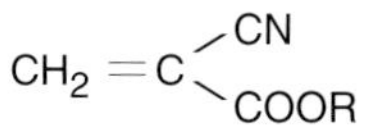

$$CH_2 = C \Big\backslash{}^{CN}_{COOR}$$

(Cyanoacrylate monomer)

If R = CH_3 $\rightarrow$ Methyl-2-cyanoacrylate
R = C_2H_5 $\rightarrow$ Ethyl-2-cyanoacrylate
R = C_4H_9 $\rightarrow$ Butyl-2-cyanoacrylate
R = $CH_3CH(CH_3)_2$ $\rightarrow$ Isobutyl-2-cyanoacrylate
R = C_8H_{17} $\rightarrow$ Octyl-2-cyanoacrylate

■ FIGURE 3–1   Basic chemical structure of the cyanoacrylate adhesives.

to certain tissue (moist or alkaline), will result in rapid polymerization and can cause significant heat during polymerization.[9,10] Short-chain monomers also degrade faster. The faster a compound degrades, the greater the amount of breakdown products (formaldehyde and cyanoacetate). In large quantities, these breakdown products can be histotoxic.[11] Formaldehyde and cyanoacetate have the potential to be cytotoxic, cause inflammatory reactions, and impair wound healing. However. in general, even the short-chain monomers, if used topically, degrade slowly enough that breakdown products are minimal before they slough off.

Longer-chain monomers, particularly four-carbon chain and longer, have been found to be optimal for clinical uses. The polymer degrades by hydrolysis, and the longer the alkyl chain, the more hydrophobic the polymer becomes. The alkyl chain of the octyl polymer is so long and hydrophobic that it can take years to degrade.[12,13] The degradation products from the longer-chain compounds are barely detectable on extraction studies. Thus, it is not surprising that the longer-chain monomers have passed International Standards Organization (ISO) standards for a nontoxic topical medical device. The low reactivity of these compounds also is accompanied by a slow polymerization process, resulting in longer setting times. In some clinical settings (topical wound closure), longer-chain compounds such as octylcyanoacrylate need an accelerator to polymerize in a clinically useful time period. This is particularly true if the formulation has had stabilizers added to it to improve stability during sterilization and to improve shelf life. Thus, it is not uncommon to have formulations of the same alkyl side chain length that have markedly different setting times.

The length and structure of the alkyl side chain also impart other important physical properties to the monomer, such as flexibility. In general, the longer or more complex (eg, octyl, methoxypropyl) the side chain, the more flexible the monomer. Physical properties become very important when one is considering the indication for the adhesive. For example, when used for topical wound closure, increased flexibility helps prevent premature sloughing of the adhesive by combating the shear forces on the interface between the adhesive and the skin (Figures 3–2 and 3–3).

MONOMERS AND FORMULATIONS

Some products contain only a monomer. The monomer polymerizes to give the adhesive strength, but other components can be added to the monomer to produce a formulation with desired properties for the intended application. These components, despite not contributing to the polymer strength, can improve clinical tensile strength by improving flexibility, viscosity, and setting times. For example, octylcyanoacrylate polymerizes far too slowly on its own, so an accelera-

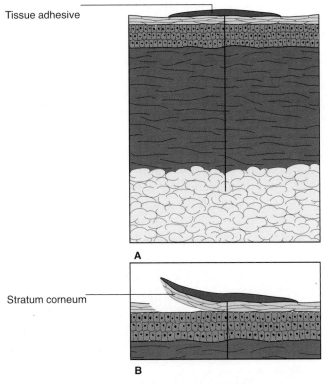

■ FIGURE 3–2   *A* and *B*, The adhesive usually sloughs off with the outermost layer of the epithelium, the stratum corneum, at 7 to 14 days. Dynamic forces cause a shearing effect, which can lead to premature sloughing.

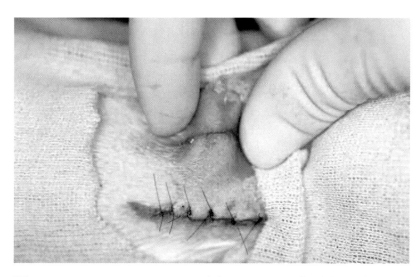

■ FIGURE 3–3   Guinea pig wound demonstrating flexibility. The octyl-cyanoacrylate formulation Dermabond has unique flexible properties that improve its tensile strength.

tor has been added to the tip of the Dermabond applicator so that the flexible properties of the monomer can be taken advantage of. The monomer becomes activated as it moves through the pores of the tip to give a desired setting time and provide a flexible topical wound closure. Similarly, when the material is too runny, adding a viscosifying agent can thicken it. Commercial superglues often use silica to form a gel. Recently, medical products have tended to viscosify the monomer by dissolving polymer back into the monomer. By incorporating flexible viscosifying agents and adding nontoxic plasticizers, one can use shorter-chain cyanoacrylate monomers in formulations and overcome their brittleness. Thus, in some instances, a formulated butyl or hexyl monomer may become as flexible as an octyl monomer yet, because of their faster polymerization qualities, would not need an accelerator.

SYNTHESIS

Cyanoacrylate adhesives are formed by combining formaldehyde and cyanoacetate in the presence of a base to form a low-molecular-weight polymer. When placed in a vacuum with heat, it becomes a liquid monomer (Figure 3–4). As manufacturing methods have become more sophisticated, it is now possible to produce a single pure monomer with few by-products. This is important when trying to produce a compound with reproducible properties and consistent performance.

POLYMERIZATION

The cyanoacrylate monomer will start to polymerize in the presence of basic substances, namely those with hydroxyl ions, such as skin moisture, water, and blood, thus bonding with skin. The process is an exothermic reaction, giving off heat in the process (Figure 3–5A). The amount of heat generated is directly related to the speed of polymerization and the amount of adhesive. The speed of polymerization is, in turn, affected by the amount of free hydroxyl ions present, the chemical structure of the cyanoacrylate adhesive, and additives such as viscosifying agents and stabilizers. The cyanoacrylate monomer consists of three parts: the cyano group, the alkyl group, and the acrylate group (Figure 3–5B). The ethylene part of the acrylate group is responsible for the polymerization. The cyano and distal alkyl portions of the alkyl-acrylate compound are highly electronegative; they polarize the carbons in the ethylene group. In the presence of a weak base, these polarized ethylene groups begin to polymerize.

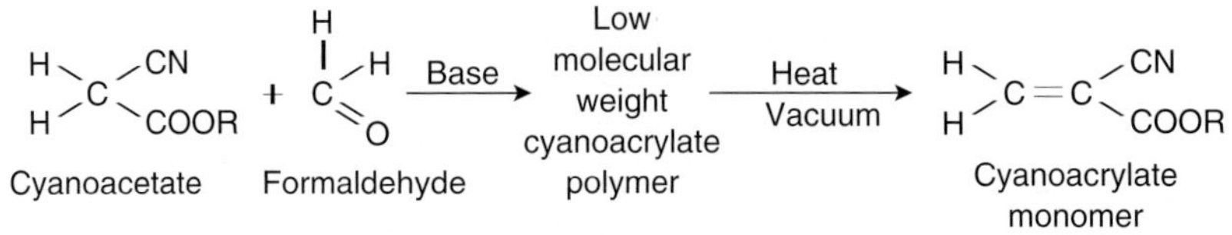

FIGURE 3–4 Synthesis of the cyanoacrylate monomer.

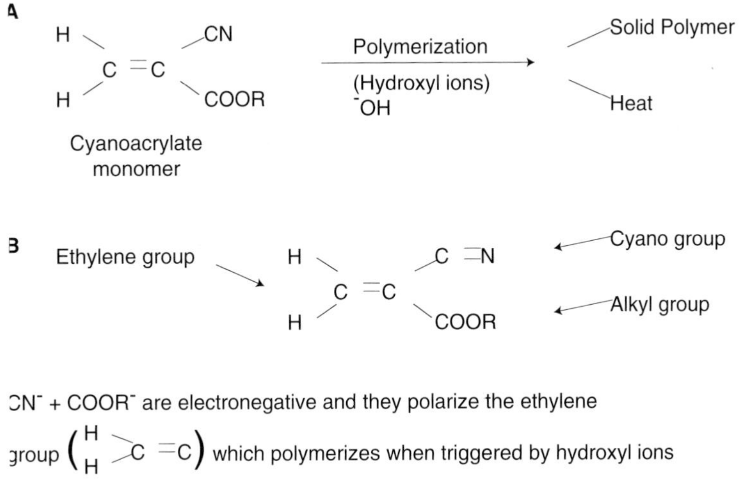

A

$$H \diagdown \qquad \diagup CN$$
$$C = C$$
$$H \diagup \qquad \diagdown COOR$$

Cyanoacrylate
monomer

Polymerization ⟶

(Hydroxyl ions)
⁻OH

Solid Polymer

Heat

B

Ethylene group ⟶

$$H \diagdown \qquad \diagup C = N$$
$$C = C$$
$$H \diagup \qquad \diagdown COOR$$

⟵ Cyano group

⟵ Alkyl group

CN⁻ + COOR⁻ are electronegative and they polarize the ethylene

group $\left(\begin{array}{c} H \\ H \end{array} \diagup C = C \right)$ which polymerizes when triggered by hydroxyl ions

■ **FIGURE 3–5** *A and B,* Polymerization of the cyanoacrylate monomer.

DEGRADATION

The degradation of the cyanoacrylate polymer occurs by hydrolysis (Figure 3–6). The straight alkyl chain derivatives are more hydrophobic depending on the length of the alkyl chain, and for the longer-chain butyl and octyl derivatives, hydrolysis may take months to years.[12,13] The breakdown products (formaldehyde and alkylcyanoacetate) can be histotoxic at high concentrations and can be absorbed cutaneously.[14] The presence of these substances is minimal when longer-chain monomers are used topically because the adhesive sloughs off after 10 to 14 days. The very-short-chain derivatives degrade faster, giving off by-products at a significantly higher concentration. This, in combination with the toxic by-products of a non-medicinal manufacturing process, may cause minor skin irritation and inflammatory responses and impair wound healing. For this reason, short-chain cyanoacrylates available commercially as superglues should not be used as medical devices.[15]

If cyanoacrylate adhesives become absorbed or implanted by accident or choice, they will be broken down internally and excreted in the urine and from the lung (see Figure 3–6).[11,12,16] Any local inflammatory response is dictated not only by the length of the alkyl side chain but also by the site of implantation (worse in vascular areas) and quantity of material used.[3]

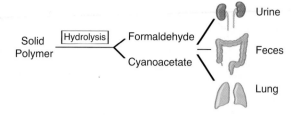

■ FIGURE 3–6   Degradation of the cyanoacrylate polymer.

ANTIMICROBIAL EFFECTS OF CYANOACRYLATE ADHESIVES

Tissue adhesives are unique in that they have antimicrobial proper-ties, especially against gram-positive organisms (Figure 3–7).[17–19] They have been shown to have lower infection rates than sutures in a contaminated wound model, although their topical use is most likely responsible for this lower infection rate.[20] The mechanism of this antimicrobial effect is unknown. Initially, the effect was thought to be due to the breakdown products formaldehyde and cyanoac-etate; however, it would be expected that smaller-chain cyanoacry-lates would have larger zones because they break down faster, giving a larger concentration of these products. However, long-chain monomers with negligible breakdown products also have a signifi-cant zone of inhibition. These zones can be as great as penicillin and cefazolin when compared on standard disk sensitivities.[18] Although the exact mechanism of this antimicrobial effect is unknown, it is postulated that polymerization leaves a highly negatively charged compound that interacts with the positively charged proteins on the cell wall of bacteria.

SAFETY, TOXICITY, AND CARCINOGENIC RISKS

Longer-chain cyanoacrylate tissue adhesives, namely butyl and octyl formulations, have been used safely on millions of patients, with no

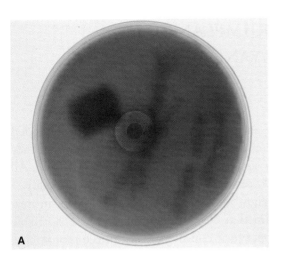
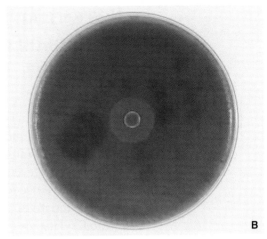

■ FIGURE 3–7   *A* and *B*, Octylcyanoacrylate and butylcyanoacrylate have an antimicrobial effect against gram-positive organisims, as demonstrated by these disk sensitivities.

reported carcinogenicity in humans. This was detailed in a study commissioned to determine any carcinogenic potential in 1986.[4] With the increased use of cyanoacrylate tissue adhesives since then, there are now numerous reported uses of cyanoacrylate adhesives in humans, without any report of carcinogenicity. One study done in the 1980s in which a large dose of the n-2-butyl monomer was injected subcutaneously into rats reported the subsequent development of sarcomas.[21] The validity and relevance of these findings are questionable for several reasons. First, the compound formulation was not designed for implantation. Second, the doses used were 100 times greater than those used in humans. Third, rats develop sarcomas quite easily when subjected to any foreign body, the so-called Oppenheimer response (rats develop a bizarre response to implanted foreign bodies that are not sufficiently porous).[22–25] Finally, the breakdown products of formaldehyde and cyanoacetate, although histotoxic in large concentration, are not in themselves carcinogenic. Attempts to reproduce or elicit any other carcinogenic response in other animals have not been reported. n-2-Butylcyanoacrylate tissue adhesive has been used topically and even implanted in millions of humans over the years, without other reports or suggestion of carcinogenicity.[26,27]

Potential for Implantable, Absorbable Cyanoacrylate Adhesives

Although cyanoacrylate adhesives are not currently recommended for implantation and use in deep tissues, this does not mean that they may not be indicated for some surgical procedures in the future. All cyanoacrylates eventually degrade and are absorbed by the body.[12] They can give rise to foreign-body reactions, as can all deep sutures. Current initiatives are aimed at developing implantable, absorbable cyanoacrylates or cyanoacrylate copolymers with no histotoxicity, causing minimal tissue reactivity and allowing for normal wound healing and tissue regeneration.

Clinical Uses

Physicians have been looking for a tissue adhesive to aid them not only for wound closure but also for other procedures.[28] They have not only tried to repair lacerations and incisions with tissue adhesives but also have attempted to use adhesives in areas in which it is difficult or nearly impossible to use sutures. Reported uses include skin, cartilage, and bone grafting; tympanoplasty and ossiculoplasty in otologic surgery; as a sealant for cerebrospinal fluid leaks and for bowel and vascular anastomosis; as an embolizing agent for arteriovenous malformations and gastric and esophageal varices; as a periodontal dressing and temporary dental sealant; as a hemostatic agent in visceral injuries; as a dressing for burns, abrasions, and blisters; and as a delivery vehicle for chemotherapeutic agents and antibiotics.[29–40] They have also been used as a temporary sealant for injured teeth with exposed nerve endings and for aphthous ulcers.[37,41–43]

The use of cyanoacrylate tissue adhesives for conditions other than topical wound closure is related mainly to regulatory approval, which varies around the world.

CYANOACRYLATES FOR TOPICAL WOUND CLOSURE

Cyanoacrylate tissue adhesives have been studied extensively compared with sutures and other wound closure agents for topical wound closure and have consistently been shown to produce similar cosmetic results while improving the speed of closure and being overall less painful.[44–50]

Suturing is a technical skill in which many physicians never develop any proficiency, whereas others suture so infrequently that they lose proficiency. Similarly, the application of a tissue adhesive is a technical skill that requires some instruction and practice to develop proficiency. Tissue adhesives are easy to learn and can easily be incorporated into a physician's practice.[51,52] However, modifications such as increasing the viscosity and improved applicator precision will make it easier for physicians to use.[53]

WOUND HEALING: IMPLICATION FOR CYANOACRYLATE TISSUE ADHESIVES

Understanding the basic concepts of wound healing is fundamental to developing an approach to using cyanoacrylates for wound closure. By understanding how wounds heal, one can appreciate why wounds in different areas of the body behave differently, require different methods of wound closure, and are subject to different rates of wound infection and cosmetic outcomes.

Physiology of Wound Healing

In the healing wound, the only structure that truly regenerates is the epithelium; the rest of the wound heals by filling in with collagen or scar tissue. There are several well-documented, orderly events that occur as a wound heals. Some of these events occur simultaneously.[54–56]

Inflammatory Phase

Immediately after a wound is closed, coagulation occurs, and cellular mediators from platelets (platelet-releasing factors) initiate a response from inflammatory cells, such as neutrophils and macrophages. These cells enter the wound to clean it up by secreting proteolytic enzymes and ingesting microorganisms and cellular debris. There is also an increase in vascular and cellular permeability at this time to allow the migration of the inflammatory cells and the cleansing of debris in the wound. This initial inflammatory response may cause redness, pain, swelling, and warmth around the wound that can be hard to distinguish from infection. It is essential that this response occur because the wound needs to be cleaned before it can heal. The inflammatory response occurs between 0 and 5 days (Figure 3–8). It is shorter in vascular areas of the body.[54]

Epithelial Phase

Epithelial cells are the only cells that regenerate during wound healing, and this process begins immediately after the wound has been closed. Shortly after wound closure, basal cells move across and down into the incised or lacerated dermis to seal off the approximated wound, protecting it from surface contamination.[57] This bar-

Inflammatory and epithelial phase

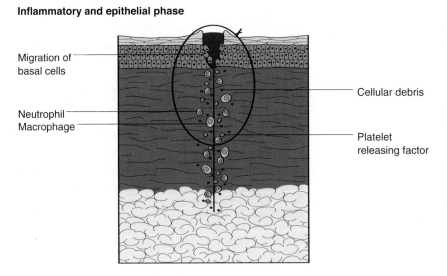

Migration of basal cells

Cellular debris

Neutrophil
Macrophage

Platelet releasing factor

■ FIGURE 3–8   The inflammatory and epithelial phase of wound healing occurs immediately and lasts up to 5 days.

rier to outside elements is formed within 48 hours, after which the fibroblast phase begins; however, until this time, the injured tissue has little or no tensile strength and is solely dependent on the wound closure device to maintain its integrity.

Fibroblast Phase

Fibroblasts are fibrous tissue germ cells that multiply rapidly, bridging the wound edges and restoring continuity. The fibroblast phase may occur as early as 48 hours after injury (Figure 3–9). Fibroblasts are stimulated by monocytes from the inflammatory phase. They synthesize and deposit collagen. Collagen is the principal structural protein of most tissues in the body. Normal tissue repair requires collagen synthesis, deposition, and cross-linking. After initial deposition, collagen is immature and gel-like in consistency. Under a series of enzymatic processes that are dependent on tissue lactate, ascorbic acid (vitamin C), and oxygen, collagen fibrils that are responsible for the strength of healing wounds are formed.[54,58,59]

Maturation Phase

Under optimal conditions, collagen production peaks in 7 days and has its greatest mass at 3 weeks. The collagen content of healing

Fibroblast phase

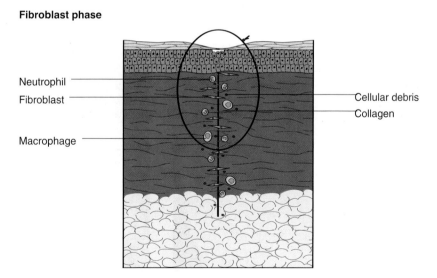

Neutrophil

Fibroblast

Macrophage

Cellular debris

Collagen

■ FIGURE 3–9   The fibroblast stage of wound healing begins as early as 48 hours after the injury.

wounds is stable after 2 months but will start to remodel itself as it mixes with fibrous tissue and improves its cross-linking (Figure 3-10). These factors alone will continue to improve the tensile strength of the wound for up to a year. As the density of collagen diminishes during this maturation phase, scars often turn pale because of decreased vascularity (Figure 3–11).[60]

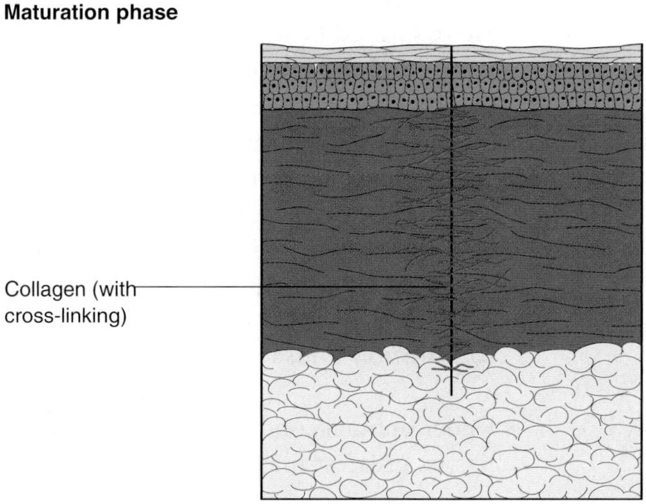

Maturation phase

Collagen (with cross-linking)

FIGURE 3-10   During the maturation stage of wound healing, collagen will remodel and mature for up to 1 year.

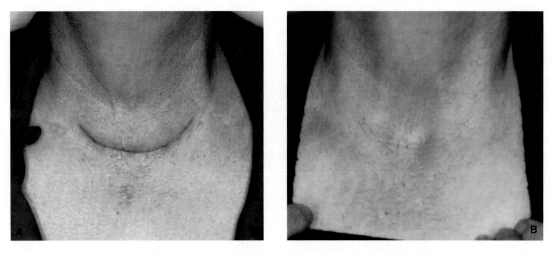

FIGURE 3–11   As a scar matures, it fades and becomes pale. *A*, Incision at 1 month. *B*, Same incision at 1 year.

Tensile Strength of Healing Wounds

After 2 days, despite epithelial growth, the wound has minimal tensile strength. After 10 days, it will have only 5 to 10% of its tensile strength and by 3 weeks, only 15 to 20%. The tensile strength will continue to improve to 60% at 4 months and can almost achieve the tensile strength of intact skin after 1 to 2 years (Figure 3–12). Wounds closed under tension develop tensile strength more quickly.[59,61]

By understanding how wound healing occurs, one can understand why using the term "glue" to describe using cyanoacrylate tissue adhesive is misleading, at best, because it implies an improper method of application. It is not surprising that when physicians hear the term "wound glue," most think of sticking the edges of the wound together just as they would glue any two objects together, as when using commercial cyanoacrylates such as Krazy Glue. In fact, putting cyanoacrylates into the wound and "gluing" the edges together was the thinking of early investigators in the 1960s and early 1970s. When used this way, tissue adhesives had a tremendous early wound-breaking strength (better than sutures), but this advantage quickly paled as inflammatory reactions and wound dehiscences occurred over the next 24 to 48 hours.[2] It was evident that cyanoacrylate tissue adhesives cannot and should not be used in this way. When

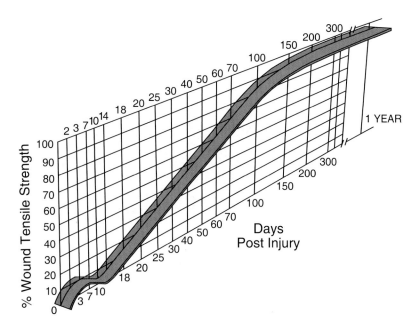

■ FIGURE 3–12 The tensile strength of a healing wound increases over time.

implanted, they trigger abnormal responses in the inflammatory phase and act as a barrier to normal epithelialization and basal cell migration, impairing the normal phases of wound healing (Figure 3–13). When complications with adhesives occur, they are commonly due to improper use. In general, improperly applied adhesive inadvertently seeps between poorly approximated wound edges, acting as a barrier to wound healing.[62] Thus, it is important that higher-viscosity formulations and improved applicators are developed to prevent this inadvertent seepage and that clinicians learn the proper indications and application techniques to avoid getting adhesive between the wound edges.

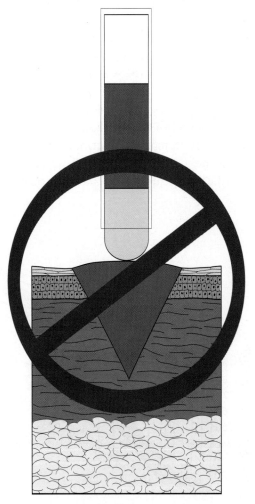

■ FIGURE 3–13   When applied between the wound edges, the adhesive acts as a barrier to normal epithelialization and, as a foreign body, impairs wound healing.

In the future, an adhesive that could be porous and/or allow healing across the material would be ideal; the tensile strength of the adhesive would be maximized, but no such adhesive currently exists. Currently, cyanoacrylate adhesives are recommended as topical agents that bond to the top layer of epithelium, the stratum corneum, and hold apposed wound edges together. Although this is not the optimal way to use the adhesive, strong, flexible cyanoacrylate adhesive formulations have been developed to form a strong topical bridge over the apposed skin edges of lacerations and incisions that can hold them together for up to 7 to 14 days. During this time, normal wound healing occurs under the adhesive (Figure 3–14). When used topically, tissue adhesives allow for normal wound healing, with no differences occurring in the tensile strength or the histologic characteristics compared with healing sutured wounds.[20,63,64]

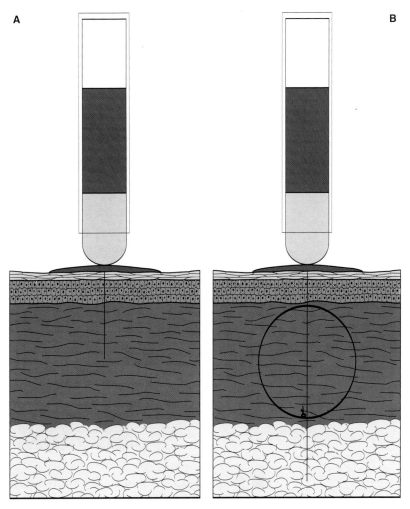

■ **FIGURE 3–14** *A and B,* The proper topical application of the tissue adhesive allows for normal wound healing to occur under the adhesive.

The breaking strength of the topical octylcyanoacrylate tissue adhesives is determined by the forces that cause shearing of the stratum corneum from the epithelium, causing a substrate failure (Figure 3-15). Because this shearing force is the limiting factor, it is unlikely that a topical adhesive could have more benefit without penetrating deeper into the epidermis or dermis, and this itself may cause more toxicity. Dynamic forces enhancing this shearing effect occur over areas of movement, such as hands and joints, and are worsened by soaking and washing. This explains the recommendations for areas in which tissue adhesives may be used or should be avoided (Table 3-1. It has been shown, however, that if areas of the body are splinted, thereby decreasing the dynamic tensile forces on the wounds, these indications may be expanded.[65]

Octylcyanoacrylate has been reported to have the greatest clinical tensile strength among the available tissue adhesives and a broader indi-

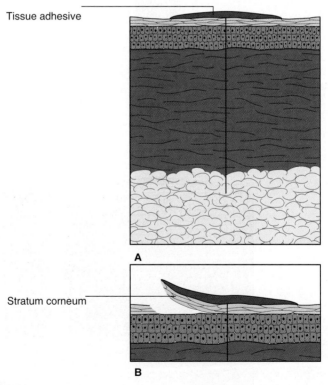

Tissue adhesive

A

Stratum corneum

B

■ FIGURE 3–15   *A* and *B*, The adhesive usually sloughs off with the outermost layer of the epithelium, the stratum corneum, at 7 to 14 days. Dynamic forces cause a shearing effect, which can lead to premature sloughing.

Table 3–1 Indications and Contraindications for Tissue Adhesives

Location	Octylcyanoacrylate	Butylcyanoacrylate
Face	All cutaneous closures	Linear lacerations < 4 cm
Lips/mucosa	No	No
Extremities	Cutaneous closure Dermal sutures recommended	Not recommended
Hand	Minor lacerations only	Not recommended
Torso	Cutaneous closure	Not recommended Dermal sutures recommended

cation for clinical use.[66] This has more to do with its flexible properties than its absolute tensile strength of the monomer (see Figure 3–3). In fact, the pure butyl monomer has tighter bonds and greater pure tensile strengththan the octyl monomer. However, long alkyl chain monomers with incorporated plasticizers give certain formulations such as Dermabond (Closure Medical Corporation, Raleigh, NC) increased flexibility to combat the shearing forces on the stratum corneum. As a result these long chain formulations have greater bridging effect and increased tensile strength and are more resistant to sloughing than pure butyl monomers (Figure 3–16). However, it is not that simple to say that all butyl formulations are inferior to octyl formulations because it is possible to manipulate the butyl formulations and increase their flexibility and performance. Pure butyl monomers set quickly on contact with skin or blood and have the advantage of not having to use an initiator during its application. Pure butyl monomers are also low viscosity and are applied as drops of glue on the wound. When the pure monomer polymerizes, a brittle bridge develops, which can easily fracture, giving it less clinical tensile strength compared with the octyl monomer (see Figure 3–16). The butyl formulations that take on the properties of octyl have incorporated flexible viscosifying agents and plasticizers. New high-viscosity products will likely consist of a combination of either octyl + butyl monomers or a pure hexyl monomer in combination with viscosifying agents and plasticizers. Optimally, this adhesive would not need an initiator (avoiding heat and applicator issues) and would take on the viscosity of honey or syrup, thus preventing the inadvertent seepage into the wounds or running onto unwanted areas.

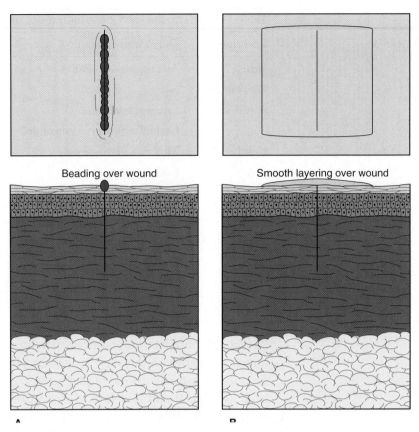

Beading over wound   Smooth layering over wound

FIGURE 3-16 *A*, Butyl beading, and *B*, octyl layering. The butyl-cyanoacrylates form a thin, narrow bridge over the wound compared with octylcyanoacrylate, which is layered on and has a wide area of application. This wider bridging action also contributes to its increased tensile strength.

PROPER WOUND CARE AND WOUND SELECTION FOR TISSUE ADHESIVES

Regardless of whether one decides to close a wound with tissue adhesive or sutures, proper wound care and evaluation are important. There have been far too many instances in which practitioners have closed wounds with tissue adhesives without proper wound care and evaluation and, as a result, have had poor outcomes, by either infections or dehiscences. There are numerous texts and references on wound care and wound healing. Below is an overview of important concepts.

History and Physical Examination

A good history should reveal the mechanism, degree of contamination, presence of a foreign body, timing of the wound, and related patient factors. Traumatic lacerations can be incised (on glass or sharp objects) or are most commonly caused by blunt objects, which produce shearing forces.[67] The extent of the trauma to the tissue should be determined. Lacerations caused by a blunt or crushing mechanism have more devitalized tissue and are at higher risk of infection.[68] All traumatic lacerations are also contaminated to some extent, making their infection rates higher than those seen in surgical incisions, but this rate is also variable depending on location. Differences in contamination, dynamic and static wound tensions, and blood flow in different regions of the body can affect outcomes. Wounds in moist areas of the body tend to be heavily colonized and subject to greater contamination and increased risk of infection.[69] Wounds in highly vascular areas heal faster and are less likely to become infected.[70,71] As a result, wounds on the face may be closed in up to 24 hours, whereas those on the hand and feet have much higher rates after 6 hours. The patient's history should reveal potential problems that may impair wound healing. The extremes of age, diabetes mellitus, immunosuppressive drugs such as steroids, chronic renal failure, obesity, and malnutrition increase the risk of a poor outcome. Allergies to anesthetics, latex, and antibiotics should be ascertained, as should the patient's tetanus status. Patients should receive immunizations in accordance with the recommendations made by the US Centers for Disease Control and Prevention (Table 3–2).

Table 3–2 Guidelines for Tetanus Prophylaxis

History of Immunization	Clean Minor Wounds		All Other Wounds	
	TD	TIG	TD	TIG
< 3 doses or uncertain ± 3 doses	Yes	No	Yes	Yes
Last dose < 5 yr	No	No	No	No
Last dose 5–10 yr	No	No	Yes	No
Last dose > 10 yr	Yes	No	Yes	No

TD = tetanus and diphtheria toxoid; TIG = tetanus immune globulin.

The wound should be examined both before and after anesthesia. Before anesthesia, the wound is examined to ascertain the neurologic and vascular functions of the injured body part distal to the injury. The neurologic function can be determined with a sensory examination, detailing two-point sensation and light touch. A motor examination will determine the strength and integrity of the tendons and muscles of the affected body part. After anesthesia, the wound should be explored carefully again for foreign bodies, the presence of tendon or muscle lacerations, underlying fractures, and/or vascular injury. When a fracture or foreign body is suspected, radiologic examination and ultrasonography can be helpful.[72]

Wound Anesthesia

There are two types of anesthesia, topical and injectable. Even for situations in which tissue adhesives are being considered, I recommend using some anesthetic (preferably topical) to allow proper examination, exploration, and hemostasis of the wound. Lidocaine and bupivacaine are the two most commonly used agents for injection (Table 3–3). Bupivacaine is longer acting and more useful when one suspects that the patient will have a persistently painful condition. Both are amide anesthetics; true anaphylactic reactions are rare because amides are incapable of forming an antigenic response. When an allergic reaction to these agents is reported, it is usually due to the methylparaben used as a preservative in the packaging. If a person reports an allergy to one of these compounds, cardiac lidocaine, which does not contain methylparaben, can be used as an alternative.[10] Injection into the affected area is a popular method of local anesthesia but can be associated with increased tissue trauma and distortion of the wound. Ideally, regional anesthesia (nerve blocks

Table 3–3 Commonly Used Injectable Local Anesthetics

Agent	Trade Name	Anesthetic Class/ Concentration	Maximum Dose, mg/kg	Duration, h
Lidocaine with epinephrine	Xylocaine	Amide 0.5–2%	5 7	1–2 2–4
Bupivacaine with epinephrine	Marcaine	Amide 0.125–0.25%	2 3	4–8 8–16

and field blocks) should be used when possible. The pain of injection can be lessened by warming and alkalinizing the anesthetic solution with sodium bicarbonate and injecting slowly; however, the clinical benefit should be weighed against time and cost because the clinical significance of the pain relief is debatable.[73,74]

Various forms of topical agents, tetracaine, adrenaline, and cocaine (TAC), as well as lidocaine, epinephrine, and tetracaine (LET), have been tried; in some cases, they can obviate the need for injectable anesthesia and the associated pain.[75] Experimental models suggest that the eutectic mixture of local anesthetics (EMLA) cream should not be used in lacerations; however, it has been used successfully in clinical situations.[76,77] The use of cocaine-containing solutions should be avoided in children when the wound is around the mucous membranes.[78]

My choice for a topical anesthetic agent is LET solution. It is easily prepared by one's local hospital pharmacy, is cheap and free of cocaine, and can be safely applied to wounds at triage by soaking a gauze bandage and having the patient or parent hold it on the area. Most wounds in areas of high vascularity (face or scalp) will need no further anesthesia even if suturing is required.[75] The anesthetic provides hemostasis and adequate anesthesia for exploration and irrigation when tissue adhesives are used. For wounds on the extremities and trunk, it can decrease the pain of injection of local anesthetics needed to supplement the anesthetic effect. Adequate anesthesia is evident when the area around the wound becomes blanched secondary to the epinephrine in the solution. The final product contains lidocaine 4%, racemic epinephrine 0.225% (equivalent to 0.1225% epinephrine), and tetracaine 0.5%. A 200 mL bottle can be made by mixing 40 mL of 20% injectable lidocaine, 20 mL of 2.25% racemic epinephrine, 50 mL of 2% tetracaine, and 90 mL of sterile water. Sodium metabisulfite (126 mg) is added to increase the stability and shelf life. A 200 mL bottle lasts 26 weeks refrigerated and 4 weeks unrefrigerated.[79]

Wound Cleansing

The area around the wound should be decontaminated and cleaned. Hair should be removed from around the wound margins to avoid contamination and entrapment. However, removal of hair from a wide area is not required. Shaving should be avoided because it can damage the hair follicles and increase the chances of infection. Long hair can be held back with gel.[80] The area around the wound can be cleaned and decontaminated with an antibacterial preparatory solution. The most common of these solutions are proviodine and chlorhexidine. These solutions, as well as hydrogen peroxide, are cytotoxic. Although they may be useful for débriding infected wounds and abscesses, they should not be used directly on or in clean wounds because they are harmful to wound healing.[81,82] Tap water or saline pressure irrigation of wounds is the most important step in wound cleansing. Because all traumatic wounds are contaminated, irrigation will decrease bacterial colonization to a level that is not infectious and should occur for most wounds, with perhaps the exception of clean facial wounds.[83] Tap water irrigation has been shown to be a cheap and efficacious method to decrease colonization owing to its high volume and pressure.[84–86] Antibiotic irrigation solutions are more expensive than sterile saline or tap water and have no added clinical benefit.[87] If tap water irrigation is impractical, sterile saline or water irrigation with a 35 cc syringe attached to an 18-gauge plastic catheter or splash guard produces optimal irrigation pressures without traumatizing healthy tissue or imbedding contaminants.[88] Splash guards are recommended to avoid the splatter of bloodborne viruses (Figure 3–17).[24] The amount of and need for irrigation should be based on the site and extent of contamination. Clean wounds in the vascular areas of the face require minimal irrigation, whereas heavily colonized wounds in areas with poor blood flow, such as bite wounds on the hands and feet, require extensive irrigation to decrease colonization rates.

Wound Tension

Assessment of wound tension is critical to assessing whether topical tissue adhesives can be used to close a wound. Wound edges should be easily approximated, and tensile shear forces should not be so great that they cause premature sloughing. There are two types of forces to consider. Immediate tensile forces on a wound may cause dehiscence, whereas prolonged forces can cause an esthetically unpleasant scar.[89,90] Wounds on different areas of and orientation to the body are subject to different tensile forces. There are two types of forces that affect the tension on the wound. Static or motionless forces are continuous owing to the depth and orientation of the wound relative to the natural tension lines of the skin (Figure 3–18). Wounds perpendicular to these tension lines are subject to greater static tensile forces. Dynamic forces owing to movement are usually obvious; moving parts, such as the hands, feet, and joints, are subject to great dynamic forces. The face and torso are less affected, but deep wounds through muscle can cause them to open when they contract.

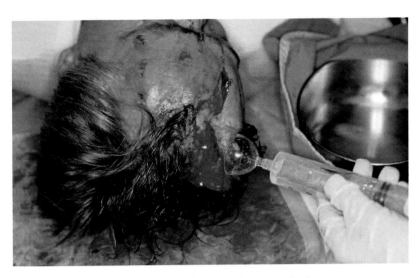

■ FIGURE 3–17   Irrigation with a splash guard device.

A good example of this is the frontalis muscle of the forehead.

Areas in which topical tissue adhesives have been successful are areas of the body under low tension and/or areas with tension removed by deep dermal sutures.

Tension on the wound will cause the scar to widen, and this widening will continue over time. Remember that a wound has only about 10% of its tensile strength at 10 days, when most skin sutures are often removed. With the skin sutures no longer present to dissipate the tensile forces on the wound, the scar can continue to widen for up to a year.[89] It would be ideal if one could leave the skin sutures in for a prolonged period; however, this is not possible because within 5 to 10 days, basal cells start to migrate down the puncture sites of sutures, and, if not removed, the so-called "suture tracks" will develop. This is why many propose the use of deep or "dermal sutures" to take the tension off the wound and why it is wise to reinforce the wound after the sutures are removed with adhesive strips or tissue adhesives.[91,92] Tissue adhesives may have an advantage over sutures because they can stay on the skin for prolonged periods of time when used for skin closure. Tissue adhesives can be used and still offer several advantages over percutaneous sutures for skin closure when deep dermal sutures are used because they are faster to apply and can avoid follow-up visits for suture removal.[49]

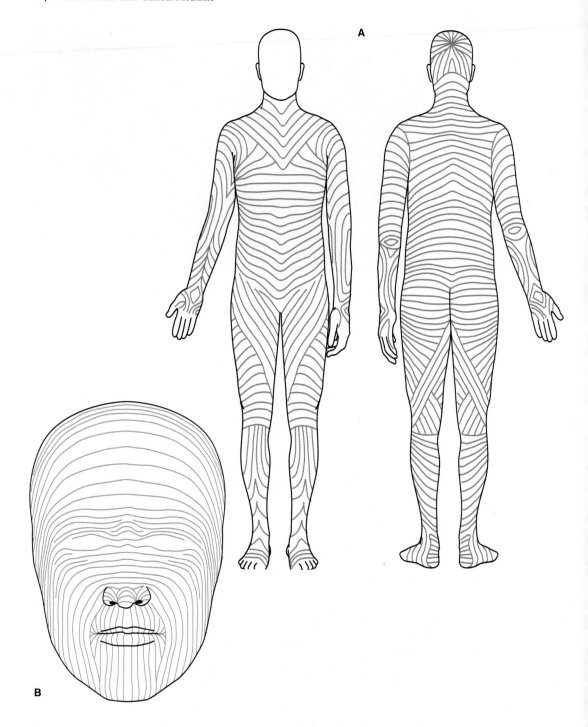

■ FIGURE 3–18 *A* and *B*, Skin tension lines on the face and body. Reproduced with permission from Brenner R, Brenner B. Emergency procedures and techniques. 2nd ed. Baltimore (MD): Williams & Wilkins.

Dermal Sutures to Relieve Tension

Wounds that are parallel to the skin tension lines and have little static tension do not require dermal sutures (Figure 3–19). Wounds perpendicular to the skin tension lines will always be difficult and have a preponderance to poor scar formation regardless of how meticulous the closure is. Any dynamic or static wound perpendicular to skin tension lines gapping greater than 5 mm requires dermal sutures. The use of dermal sutures in wounds increases infection rates.[93] On cosmetically sensitive and highly vascular areas such as the face, they are recommended as described. In areas in which cosmesis is less important, the risk of infection in contaminated wounds may prohibit their use. The correct technique for the dermal suture is shown in Figure 3–20. Three well-placed dermal sutures can take enough tension off most wounds: one midpoint and then one each between the midpoint and wound edge (Figure 3–21).

The material used for the dermal sutures should be absorbable and provide strength to the wound for the longest period of time. Therefore, plain surgical gut should be avoided because it loses most of its tensile strength in 5 to 7 days. Sutures to be considered are polyglactin, polyglycolic acid, polydixanone, and polyglyconate. The size of the dermal suture should be comparable to the size of the suture used to close skin in that area of the body.

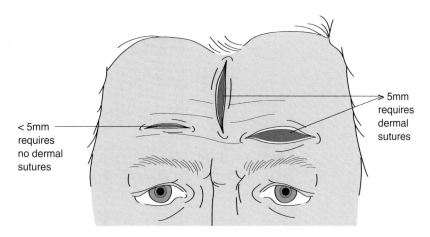

■ FIGURE 3–19 Wounds requiring dermal (deep) sutures on the face. Wounds under tension gapping more than 5 mm require buried dermal sutures.

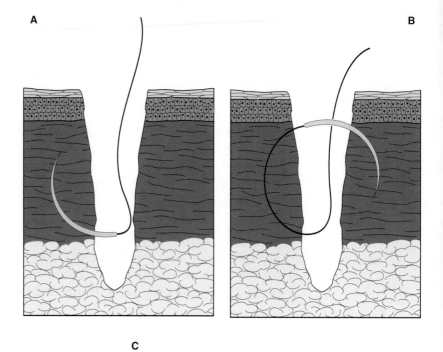

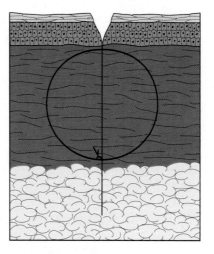

■ **FIGURE 3–20** *A* to *C,* Dermal or deep suture techniques. The suture is in the dermis, not in fat or connective tissue, and the knot is buried (*C*).

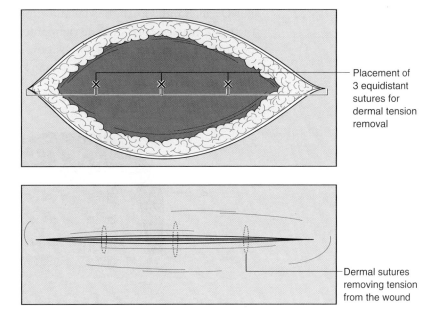

FIGURE 3–21 *A* and *B*, Placement of dermal sutures. Three well-placed dermal sutures can take the tension off most wounds.

Proper Application of Tissue Adhesives for Topical Wound Closure

1. Provide appropriate wound care techniques.
2. Where possible, use topical anesthetics with vasoconstrictive properties to improve hemostasis and allow proper exploration and irrigation.
3. Make sure the laceration or incision is appropriate for the use of the tissue adhesive formulation that you plan to use. Pure butyl monomers have excellent clinical outcomes but, because of their brittleness, have fewer clinical indications. Use dermal sutures where appropriate (see Table 3–1).
4. Ensure that the patient or wound is on a horizontal plane. Most tissue adhesives have a low viscosity, and there may be runoff in gravity-dependent areas (Figure 3–22).
5. Acquire hemostasis (pressure or epinephrine-containing topical anesthetics).
6. Appose wound edges with fingers, forceps, or skin hooks (Figure 3–23). Sometimes steri-strips are helpful to appose edges before applying the adhesive, and adhesive can be applied over top of them. If edges cannot be easily apposed, then an alternate method of wound closure should be considered.

7. **For Dermabond:** Crush the vial and express the adhesive through the tip. Practice expressing the right amount. Precise amounts can be applied using the higher-viscosity formulation and the precision Pro-Pen applicator and/or a snap-on tip (Figure 3–24) (see the video on the CD-ROM).

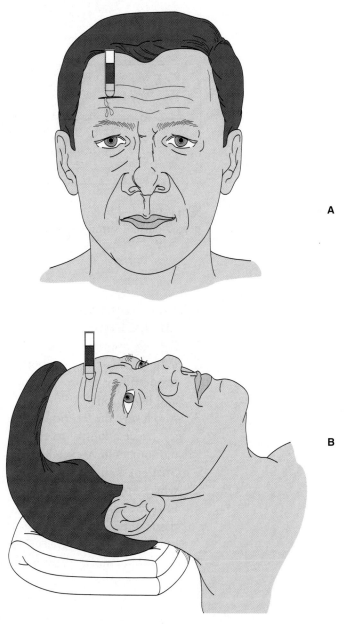

A

B

■ FIGURE 3–22   *A* and *B*, Wound positioned on a horizontal plane. The wound should be positioned on the horizontal plane to prevent the adhesive from running into unwanted areas.

Paint the adhesive over the approximated wound edges. Do not push the tip into the wound. Apply the adhesive in two to three coatings, allowing each to dry slightly before applying the next layer. If one thick layer is applied, the heat from the exothermic polymerization may cause a burning discomfort to the patient and, in some cases, a minor thermal injury (Figure 3–25). This is another reason to use a topical anesthetic. There is an optimal thickness to be applied that likely depends on the clinical site where the adhesive is used. However, the current applicator does not allow for a consistent application or precise thickness.

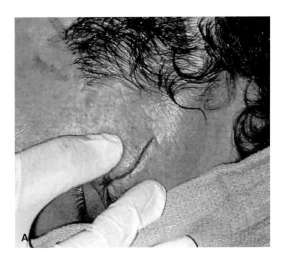
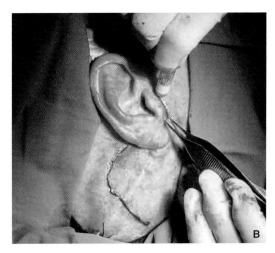

■ FIGURE 3–23   *A* and *B*, Appose wounds with fingers or forceps.

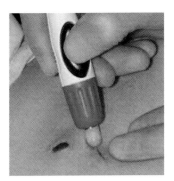

■ FIGURE 3–24   The new Pro-Pen applicator with its precision tip, along with the new high-viscosity formula, is a welcomed adjunct and will improve one's ability to apply the adhesive properly.

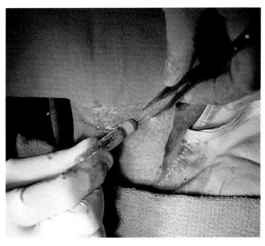

■ FIGURE 3–25   The adhesive painted over the approximated wound edges.

For Indermil or Histoacryl: Because these adhesives are quick setting and do not require an initiator, their application is different from that of Dermabond. Before opening the ampule, hold it in one hand with the tip pointed upward. Sharply flick the tip with the forefinger of the other hand to remove any adhesive trapped in the tip. While still holding the ampule in the vertical position, twist and snap off the winged cap for Indermil (United States Surgical, a Division of Tyco Healthcare Group, LP, Norwalk, CT) or cut Histoacryl (B. Braun, Melsungen AG, Melsungen, Germany) off at the hub. It is recommended to use an access canula (Indermil) (Figure 3–26) or that a 25-gauge needle (Histoacryl) (Figures 3–27 and 3–28) be attached to the vials to provide greater control during application. Do not exert excess pressure on the ampule when affixing the cannula or needle, and keep the vial upright until ready for use. Apply the tissue adhesive very sparingly, either as minute drops (spot welding) or as a very thin film along the edges of the wound (Figure 3–29). Avoid heavy application because the monomer is low viscosity and can easily run on unwanted areas.

8. Maintain apposition of the wound for 30 to 60 seconds. The polymerization time can vary based on the length of the alkyl side chain, the amount of stabilizers added to the formulation, and, if used, the amount of initiator. Drying of the adhesive usually occurs in 2 to 3 minutes (Figure 3–30).

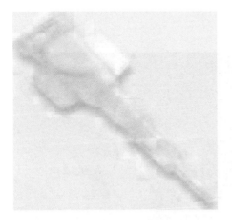

■ FIGURE 3–26 Indermil has an additional applicator tip, which is shown attached in this figure. Like the 25-gauge needle applied to the Histoacryl vial, it allows fine application of the adhesive.

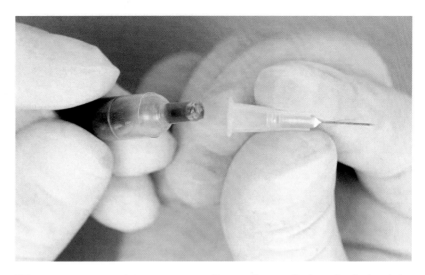

■ FIGURE 3–27   A 25-gauge needle can be applied to the hub of the Histoacryl vial to allow fine application.

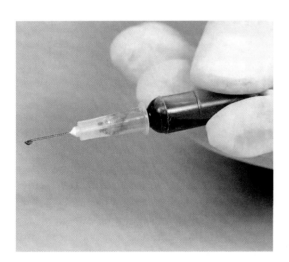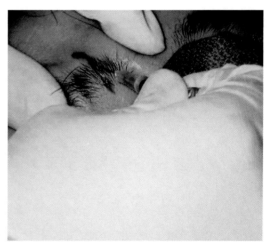

■ FIGURE 3–28   *A* and *B,* The adhesive is applied onto the wound as drops in a "spot welding" technique.

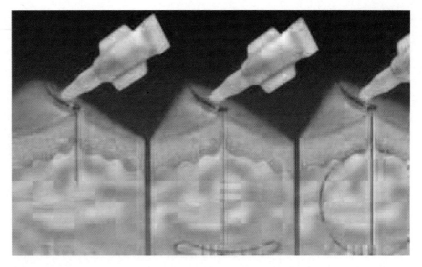

■ FIGURE 3–29 Indermil, like Histoacryl, is dropped on the surface of well-apposed wound edges in a technique often referred to as "spot welding."

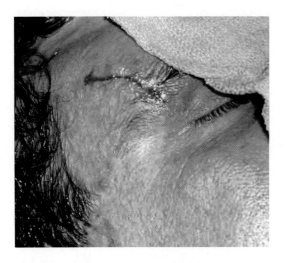

■ FIGURE 3–30 When the adhesive begins to polymerize, maintain apposition for 30 to 60 seconds. Full strength occurs at 2 minutes. After polymerization, the wound can be seen under the transparent adhesives. Sometimes, despite hemostasis, a small amount of blood will mix in with some of the adhesive, as it does at the top of the wound.

AVOIDING PITFALLS WHEN USING CYANOACRYLATES FOR WOUND CLOSURE

Complications and poor outcomes with the use of tissue adhesive can be avoided by selecting the proper wounds for closure and ensuring that the wound edges are completely apposed before application and that no adhesive gets between the wound edges.

CHOOSING THE RIGHT WOUND FOR TISSUE ADHESIVE WOUND CLOSURE

Avoiding complications by choosing the appropriate wounds for closure with tissue adhesives is most important. Skin edges must be easily apposed either manually or with deep sutures or steri-strips to be considered candidates for using tissue adhesives to close the wounds. As a rule, one should be confident that the edges of the wound can be tightly and evenly apposed with manual methods, as they would be if sutures were used.

Deep dermal sutures can be used to take the tension off the wound and make the edges easier to appose. Some have questioned using tissue adhesives when they have already placed deep sutures, but, in general, tissue adhesives that are highly flexible, such as Dermabond, can replace percutaneous monofilament sutures in these circumstances regardless of the length of the wound or incision. This prevents the need for return visits in these cases, and in these circumstances, the adhesive can provide its own wound dressing, making it cost-effective.[49]

In cases in which manual wound edge approximation is possible but awkward to maintain, one should consider using short, fine adhesive tapes to attain and maintain wound approximation while the adhesive is applied (Figure 3–31). The tissue adhesives are left in place and can also add extra reinforcement on areas such as the chin. This method also avoids the risk of low-viscosity adhesives running and sticking the surgeon's glove to the patient.

Hemostasis

Hemostasis is important in providing a neat, secure wound closure. Blood and fluids trigger polymerization. If there is an excess of these fluids, polymerization will occur too rapidly, with the adhesive bonding to the fluid and protein in the blood and not the skin. This results in the forming of an unsightly plastic mass on top of the wound, which does little to actually bond the skin. Hemostasis can be obtained with dermal sutures where appropriate; pressure on the wound or vasoconstrictor solutions (eg, 1:1,000 topical epinephrine) can be used. LET is optimal because it also has significant anesthetic properties. When applied to a properly prepared wound, the adhesive is transparent and the well-apposed edges under the adhesive can be seen (Figure 3–32).

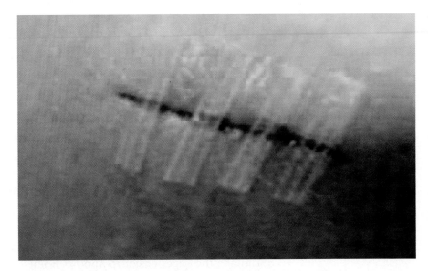

■ FIGURE 3–31   This chin laceration had the edges well approximated with steri-strips first (note that these are cut short). Tissue adhesive can then be applied on top of the steri-strips, which are left in place as added reinforcement. This technique is useful in certain areas, such as the chin, or when it is difficult to manually appose wound edges.

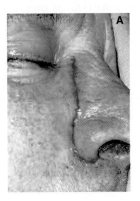
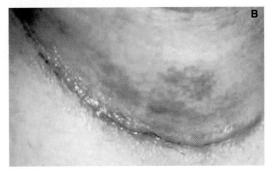

■ FIGURE 3–32   *A* and *B*, With good hemostasis and proper application, the incision line can be seen under the transparent adhesive.

Do Not Get Adhesive in the Wound!

It cannot be stressed enough that extra caution be taken to avoid putting any adhesive in the wound. The rationale is clearly explained in the wound-healing section. If the wound edges are tightly apposed, and the adhesive is painted on top of the wound, in general, the adhesive should not seep into the wound to any significant degree. Unfortunately, a common mistake is to have material inadvertently seep between the wound edges because of incomplete apposition. This is a problem especially with low-viscosity materials, which can easily seep between gaps if not drawn into them by capillary action. Although the wound may initially look good, this scenario often results in poor wound healing and late dehiscences. I believe that this is a major source of the problem when clinicians report problems (especially late dehiscences > 2 days) and poor outcomes when using tissue adhesives.[62]

Several precautions can be taken to achieve optimal results. If complete wound apposition is too difficult to achieve, consider another closure device or adjunct to help. Often for large wounds and incisions, having an assistant use forceps is helpful, and the use of a deep dermal suture can take tension off the wound.

Another common mistake is to inadvertently deposit the adhesive into the wound by pushing the tip of the vial into the wound and separating the wound edges. The adhesive should be expressed from the tip by squeezing the vial and applied by lightly painting the adhesive over apposed edges. The adhesive should not be expressed by putting pressure on the tip (as with a marking pen). This will put pressure on the wound margins, cause the edges to invert, and deposit the adhesive into the wound (Figure 3–33).

Finally, whereas physicians need to take precautions to avoid depositing material between wound edges, manufacturers of these products need to address and are addressing the problem as well. Much of the problem lies with the crude applicators and low-viscosity adhesives that can easily seep into wounds or even be drawn in by capillary action. Original Dermabond and Indermil have viscosities around 4 to 5 cps, which are very close to that of water. Higher-viscosity adhesives will certainly help with this problem. Dermabond is now available in a higher-viscosity formula at approximately 50 cps. Although even higher viscosities are likely optimal, the changes made are a significant improvement, especially if combined with the precision tip applicator.[53] By increasing viscosity and controlling the volume and mass applied, fewer complications and better outcomes are inevitable.

Avoiding Heat

When the adhesive polymerizes, an exothermic reaction occurs and heat is liberated. The amount of heat or burning felt by patients is variable. Fifty percent of patients feel no discomfort, whereas some feel a definite burning sensation.[3] The amount of heat generated is dependent on several factors: the speed of polymerization (use of ini-

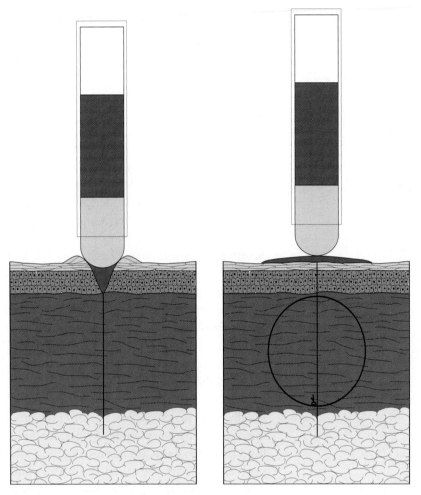

■ **FIGURE 3–33** *A* and *B*, If the applicator is pushed into the wound, it will deposit adhesive between the wound edges. The adhesive should be brushed on top of the wound.

tiators), the amount of adhesive applied, and the moisture content of the patient's skin (another reason to obtain good hemostasis). Aside from achieving hemostasis, the best way to avoid any discomfort caused by the heat is to apply the adhesive in thin layers with multiple strokes and to use topical anesthetics. This way, the first layer can act as insulation and prevent a large mass of adhesive polymerizing all at once.

Controlling the Amount of Adhesive and Runoff

Most available adhesives have a low viscosity, have a tendency to run off into unwanted areas, and can seep between wound edges that are not tightly apposed. Although higher-viscosity formulations will improve control over the application, practical steps can be taken to deal with this problem. Make sure that the part to be treated is on a horizontal plane or in the Trendelenburg position (see Figure 3–22). Position the patient such that if the adhesive runs, it will do so away from unwanted areas, such as the eye.[94] One can also control Dermabond by squeezing and releasing the vial; the amount of adhesive expressed can be controlled (when released, the adhesive on the tip will be sucked up by a vacuum mechanism). The Pro-Pen applicator takes advantage of this mechanism to allow a more precise delivery.

Erroneous Application

If the adhesive gets to an unintended place, it can usually be wiped off before it sets. If the adhesive is implanted erroneously between the wound edges, the wound should be anesthetized and débrided to remove the adhesive. If adhesive gets into the eye, it can be easily removed with ophthalmic ointment. The emollients in the ointment help break down the adhesive and soften it. It is recommended that a patch with ointment be applied over the eye for 24 hours (Figure 3–34). The adhesive can then be easily removed from the eyelashes. It should not be necessary to cut the eyelashes. If the adhesive gets on the cornea, it will simply slough off or can be removed like any foreign body. Cyanoacrylates have been used to treat many disorders of the cornea and are nontoxic.[95] On other areas, the adhesive can be removed with acetone; however, care should be taken because acetone should not be used on open wounds because of its histotoxicity.

Wound Aftercare

Tissue adhesives form their own waterproof antimicrobial dressing and do not require any additional protective dressings.[96,97] Although patients may shower after the use of tissue adhesives, they should not soak or scrub the area because this can lead to premature sloughing of the adhesive, leading to wound dehiscence. After showering, the area can be gently patted dry. Ointment should not be applied to the adhesive because ointments promote degradation and premature sloughing of the adhesive from the upper layer of skin, the stratum corneum.

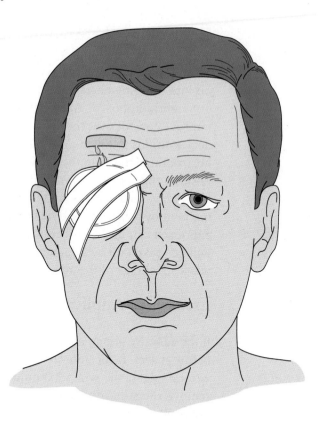

■ FIGURE 3–34   If the adhesive inadvertently gets into the eye, apply ophthalmic ointment and a patch. The ointment will soften and loosen the adhesive, allowing for easy removal after 24 hours.

COST-EFFECTIVENESS OF CYANOACRYLATES FOR TOPICAL WOUND CLOSURE

Tissue adhesives for wound closure have been studied thoroughly. No area of wound care or any wound closure device has been studied so extensively with prospective trials. Numerous trials have been done to date, and in all of these trials, there were no clinical or statistical differences in the cosmetic outcomes between traditional wound closure (mainly sutures) and tissue adhesives.[44,45,50] In most of the trials, the physicians had little experience in the use of tissue adhesives, whereas most were experienced suturers, giving any possible advantage to the traditional wound closure. In trials in which there was one experienced surgeon applying the adhesive, there has been a trend to superior results with tissue adhesives.[48,98] This demonstrates the importance of proficiency in the application of these agents. Regardless of who is applying them, there is overwhelming evidence that tissue adhesives provide as good if not better cosmetic closure for lacerations and incisions when compared to sutures.

Tissue adhesives are more cost-effective for topical skin closure than traditional percutaneous sutures that require suture removal. A physician visit for suture removal can be avoided and can significantly lower the overall cost for the closure of a laceration or incision. In addition to the convenience for the patient, parents do not need to take time off work or a busy schedule to attend the visit. For the same reason, adhesive tapes and absorbable sutures are also cost-effective. Tissue adhesive application also decreases the practitioner time to repair a wound by 10 to 15 minutes. Although this cost is often not figured into the costs of a visit, it is a real dollar amount value that should be considered because the practitioner is freed up earlier and able to generate revenue by treating other patients.

In Canada, Histoacryl Blue is supplied in a vial that is often reused. It has been reported that a vial costing $25.00 (US) can repair 8 to 10 lacerations, producing a cost of approximately $3.00 per laceration repair; however, reusing the product is not condoned. Single-dose sterile products (Dermabond and Indermil) are available at approximately $20 to $25, depending on the volume purchased. Single-dose, nonsterile, non-FDA products, such as "Glue-Stitch," sell for $6 to $8 for single use in Canada.

A formal cost analysis has been done comparing the cost of nonabsorbable percutaneous sutures, absorbable percutaneous sutures, and the tissue adhesive Histoacryl Blue for the repair of lacerations treated in an emergency department. This formal analysis was done in Canada and looked at personnel time, the cost of supplies, and parental costs. Overhead emergency department costs and complications were felt to be equal for each group and were not included in the analysis. The study showed that nonabsorbable sutures were 6.8 times more costly than the tissue adhesives. Ninety percent of patients chose tissue adhesives as their first choice of wound closure and were willing to pay a median of $40 for tissue adhesives if they were not covered by their insurance.[99]

Both the simple butyl monomer and the octyl formulation have been used successfully to close small wounds under low tension, and as newer formulations are developed and come to market, the ease of use, comfort level of the physician with the application technique, performance, and cost will be the driving forces for choosing one product over another.

CYANOACRYLATE ADHESIVES AS TOPICAL WOUND DRESSINGS OR BANDAGES

Cyanoacrylate adhesives can be applied topically to burns, abrasions, and minor cuts, with excellent results.[100] There have been reports that burns treated with cyanoacrylate have improved epithelialization and healing.[101–105] The adhesive forms a waterproof seal of the wound and provides an antimicrobial barrier.[97,106] Several different cyanoacrylate products are approved by the FDA as nonexempt class I devices as liquid bandages (Liquid Band-aid, Ethicon, Inc., Somerville, NJ; NexCare Liquid Bandage, 3M Minneapolis, MN) and are being sold directly to consumers. As these devices become easier to use (consumer-friendly applicators, higher viscosity), the advantages of liquid bandages over conventional bandages (precise application, waterproof, flexible, stay on longer, antimicrobial barrier and dressing) will likely result in tremendous growth in the consumer liquid bandage market over the next several years.

In a related use, Sooth and Seal (Closure Medical, Raleigh, NC) is a cyanoacrylate used to treat aphthous ulcers of the mouth.[42,43] Other related cyanoacrylates are becoming more popular to prevent chafing, blisters, and turf burns in athletes.

CYANOACRYLATES AS EMBOLIZATION AGENTS

Trufill n-Butyl Cyanoacrylate (n-BCA) Liquid Embolic System is a three-component system containing n-butylcyanoacrylate (n-BCA), ethiodized oil, and tantalum powder and is the first class III cyanoacrylate-associated embolic agent. Specifically, the final composition of this embolic agent is a mixture of tantalum power and ethiodized oil that is mixed with an n-BCA monomer (99.5% n-BCA with other ingredients), and it is used under fluoroscopic guidance to obstruct or reduce the blood flow to cerebral arteriovenous malformations via superselective catheter delivery.[107,108] On contact with body fluids or tissue, the mixture polymerizes into a solid material.

The ethiodized oil is a radiopaque polymerizing retardant and will vary the rate of polymerization of n-BCA. The finely ground dark gray metal tantalum powder is used to provide additional radiopacification to the n-BCA + ethiodized oil mixture. The intended use of the Trufill n-Butyl Cyanoacrylate (n-BCA) Liquid Embolic System is as an embolic agent for cerebral arteriovenous malformations. It has no other existing approvals for use in other areas of the body.

FUTURE CYANOACRYLATE TISSUE ADHESIVE PRODUCTS

The number of reported off-label uses of cyanoacrylate tissue adhesives continues to grow. Similarly, the number of FDA approvals will grow, and new tissue adhesive formulations will be developed to meet these clinical demands. Long-chain cyanoacrylate adhesives may not be the answer for internal use either as a sealant or wound closure because they take years to degrade. The answer may lay in short-chain products, which degrade rapidly but whose toxicity can be neutralized through the use of copolymers. These products would have to maintain some flexibility to suit the clinical situation. Work is being done in this area, but it will be years before a clinical product becomes available. Implantable products that have a greater porosity and allow collagen and fibroblast growth across them would be of great value in wound healing.

In the meantime, manipulation of the current cyanoacrylate tissue adhesive formulations would likely increase and improve their ease of use. Increased viscosity and improved applicators have and will improve the application and control of these adhesives, achieving better results.

Cyanoacrylate tissue adhesive technology is growing rapidly. The currently available products for wound treatment are just the tip of the iceberg. The goal of this chapter is to familiarize physicians with the technology of cyanoacrylate tissue adhesives and the proper use of the currently available products for wound closure. Hopefully, it will also serve as a foundation for understanding the new products that are likely to appear over the next several years.

REFERENCES

1. Coover HN, Joyner FB, Sheere NH. Chemistry and performance of cyanoacrylate adhesive. J Soc Plast Surg Eng 1959;15:5–6.

2. Houston S, Hodge JW Jr, Ousterhout DK, Leonard F. The effect of alpha-cyanoacrylates on wound healing. J Biomed Mater Res 1969;3:281–9.

3. Toriumi DM, Raslam WF, Freidman M, et al. Variable histotoxicity of Histoacryl when used in a subcutaneous site: an experimental study. Laryngoscope 1991;101:339–43.

4. Kung H. Evaluation of the undesirable side effects of the surgical use of Histoacryl glue with special regard to possible carcinogenicity. Basel (Switzerland): RCC Institute for Contract Research; 1986. Project 064315.

5. Keng TM, Bucknall TE. A clinical trial of tissue adhesive in skin closure of groin wounds. Med J Malaysia 1989;44:122–8.

6. Mizrahi S, Bickel A, Ben-Layish EB. Use of tissue adhesives in the repair of lacerations in children. J Pediatr Surg 1988;23:312–3.

7. Galil KA, Shofield ID, Wright GD. Effect of n-butyl-2-cyanoacrylate (Histoacryl Blue) on the healing of skin wounds. J Can Dent Assoc 1984;50:565–9.

8. Leonard F. The n-alkylalphacyanoacrylate tissue adhesives. Ann N Y Acad Sci 1968;146:203–13.

9. Matsumoto T, Hardaway RM III, Heisterkamp CA III, et al. Higher homologous cyanoacrylate tissue adhesives in surgery of internal organs. Arch Surg 1967;94:861–4.

10. Matsumoto T, Pani KC, Hardaway RM, Leonard F. n-Alkyl-alpha-cyanoacrylate monomers in surgery. Speed of polymerization and method of their application. Arch Surg 1967;94:153–6.

11. Wade CW, Leonard F. Degradation of poly(methyl 2-cyanoacrylates). J Biomed Mater Res 1972;6:215–20.

12. Pani KC, Gladieux G, Brandes G, et al. The degradation of n-butyl alpha-cyanoacrylate tissue adhesive. II. Surgery 1968;63:481–9.

13. Woodward SC, Herrman JB, Cameron JL, et al. Histotoxicity of cyanoacrylate tissue adhesive in the rat. Ann Surg 1965;162:113.

14. Ousterhout DK, Gladieux GV, Leonard F. Cutaneous absorption of n-alkyl alpha-cyanoacrylate. J Biomed Mater Res 1968;2:157–63.

15. Wang AA, Martin CH. Full-thickness skin necrosis of the fingertip after application of superglue. J Hand Surg [Am] 2003;28:696–8.

16. Ousterhout DK, Gladieux GV, Wade CW, et al. Digestive tract absorption of alkyl alpha-cyanoacrylate-beta-14-C. Oral Surg Oral Med Oral Pathol 1969;27:410–6.

17. Quinn JV, Osmond MH, Yurack JA, Moir PJ. n-2 Butylcyanoacrylate: risk of bacterial contamination with an appraisal of its antimicrobial effects. J Emerg Med 1995;13:581–5.

18. Quinn JV, Ramotar K, Osmond MH. The antimicrobial effects of a new tissue adhesive. Acad Emerg Med 1996;3:536.

19. Lehman RA, West RL, Leonard F. Toxicity of alkyl 2-cyanoacrylates. II. Bacterial growth. Arch Surg 1966;93:447–50.

20. Quinn JV, Maw JL, Ramotar K, et al. Octylcyanoacrylate tissue adhesive wound repair versus suture wound repair in a contaiminated wound model. Surgery 1997;122:69–72.

21. Reiter A. [Induction of sarcomas by the tissue-binding substance Histoacryl Blue in the rat]. Z Exp Chir Transplant Kunstliche Organe 1987;20(1):55–60.

22. Oppenheimer ET, Willhite M, Danismefski I, Stout AT. Observation of the effects of powder polymers in carcinogen production. Cancer Res 1961;21:132–4.

23. Oppenheimer BS, Oppenheimer, ET, Stout AP, et al. The latent period in carcinogenesis by plastics in rats and its relation to the presarcomatous stage. Cancer 1958;11:204–13.

24. Oppenheimer ET. Autoradiographic studies on the connective tissue pocket formed around imbedded plastics. Cancer Res 1960;20:654–7.

25. Reno FE. Carcinogenicity testing. In: Williams P, Hottendorf G, editors. Comprehensive toxicology. Oxford (UK): Elsevier Science Ltd; 1997. p. 2.

26. Matsumoto T, Heisterkamp CA III. Long-term study of aerosol cyanoacrylate tissue adhesive spray: carcinogenicity and other untoward effects. Am Surg 1969;35:825–7.

27. Matsumoto T. Carcinogenesis and cyanoacrylate adhesives. JAMA 1967;202:1057.

28. Hallock GG. Expanded applications for octyl-2-cyanoacrylate as a tissue adhesive. Ann Plast Surg 2001;46:185–9.

29. Olsson SE, Rietz KA. Polymer osteosynthesis. II. An experimental study with methyl 2- cyanoacrylate (Eastman 910 adhesive) in bone grafting. Acta Chir Scand Suppl 1966;367:4–19.

30. Kaufman RS. The use of tissue adhesive (isobutyl cyanoacrylate) and topical steroid (0.1 percent dexamethasone) in experimental tympanoplasty. Laryngoscope 1974;84:793–804.

31. Smyth GD, Kerr AG. Histoacryl (butyl cyanoacrylate) as an ossicular adhesive. J Laryngol Otol 1974;88:539–42.

32. Maw JL, Kartush JM. Ossicular chain reconstruction using a new tissue adhesive. Am J Otol 2000;21:301–5.

33. Maw JL, Kartush JM, Bouchard K, Raphael Y. Octylcyanoacrylate: a new medical-grade adhesive for otologic surgery. Am J Otol 2000;21:310–4.

34. Papadakis N, Mark VH. Repair of spinal cerebrospinal fluid fistula with the use of a tissue adhesive: technical note. Neurosurgery 1980;6:63–5.

35. Lunderquist A, Borjesson B, Owman T, Bengmark S. Isobutyl 2-cyano-acrylate (bucrylate) in obliteration of gastric coronary vein and esophageal varices. AJR Am J Roentgenol 1978;130:1–6.

36. Akers WA, Leonard F, Ousterhout DK, Cortese TA Jr. Treating friction blisters with alkyl-cyanoacrylates. Arch Dermatol 1973;107:544–7.

37. Herod EL. Cyanoacrylates in dentistry: a review of the literature. J Can Dent Assoc 1990;56:331–4.

38. Collins JA, James PM, Levitsky SA, et al. Cyanoacrylate adhesives as topical hemostatic aids. II. Clinical use in seven combat casualties. Surgery 1969;65:260–3.

39. Couvreur P. Polyalkylcyanoacrylates as colloidal drug carriers. Crit Rev Ther Drug Carrier Syst 1988;5(1):1–20.

40. Seewald S, Mendoza G, Seitz U, et al. Variceal bleeding and portal hypertension: has there been any progress in the last 12 months? Endoscopy 2003;35:136–44.

41. Jasmin JR, Muller-Giamarchi M, Jonesco-Benaiche N. Local treatment of minor aphthous ulceration in children. ASDC J Dent Child 1993;60:26–8.

42. Kutcher MJ, Ludlow JB, Samuelson AD, et al. Evaluation of a bioadhesive device for the management of aphthous ulcers. J Am Dent Assoc 2001;132:368–76.

43. Kutcher M. Evaluating the efficacy of 2-octyl cyanoacrylate bioadhesive for treatment of oral ulcerations. Compend Contin Educ Dent Suppl 2001;32:12–6.

44. Quinn JV, Wells GA, Sutcliffe T, et al. A randomized trial comparing octylcyanoacrylate tissue adhesive and sutures in the management of lacerations. JAMA 1997;277:1527–30.

45. Quinn JV, Drzewiecki A, Li MM, et al. A randomized, controlled trial comparing a tissue adhesive with suturing in the repair of pediatric facial lacerations. Ann Emerg Med 1993;22:1130–5.

46. Singer AJ, Hollander JE, Valentine SM, et al. Prospective randomized controlled trial of a new tissue adhesive (2-octylcyanoacrylate) versus standard wound closure techniques for laceration repair. Acad Emerg Med 1998;5:94–8.

47. Bruns TB, Robinson BS, Smith RJ, et al. A new tissue adhesive for laceration repair in children. J Pediatr 1998;132:1067–70.

48. Maw JL, Quinn JV, Wells GA, et al. A prospective comparison of octylcyanoacrylate tissue adhesive and sutures for the closure of head and neck incisions. J Otolaryngol 1997;26:26–30.

49. Matin SF. Prospective randomized trial of skin adhesive versus sutures for closure of 217 laparoscopic port-site incisions. J Am Coll Surg 2003;196:845–53.

50. Singer AJ, Quinn JV, Clark RE, Hollander JE. Closure of lacerations and incisions with octylcyanoacrylate: a multicenter randomized

controlled trial. Surgery 2002;131:270–6.

51. Hollander JE, Singer AJ. Application of tissue adhesive: rapid attainment of proficiency. Acad Emerg Med 1998;5:1012–7.

52. Lin M, Coates WC, Lewis RJ. Tissue adhesive skills study: the physician learning curve. Pediatr Emerg Care 2004;20:219–23.

53. Singer AJ, Giordano P, Fitch JL, et al. Evaluation of a new high-viscosity octylcyanoacrylate tissue adhesive for laceration repair: a randomized, clinical trial. Acad Emerg Med 2003;10:1134–7.

54. Hunt TK. The physiology of wound healing. Ann Emerg Med 1988;17:1274.

55. Hunt TK, Van Winkle W Jr. Normal repair. In Hunt TK, editor. Fundamentals of wound management. New York: Appleton-Century-Croft; 1979.

56. Jackson DS, Rovee DT. Current concepts in wound healing: research and theory. J Enterostom Ther 1988;15:133.

57. Schauerhamer RA, Edlich RF, Panek P, et al. Studies in the management of the contaminated wound. VII. Susceptibility of surgical wounds to postoperative surface contamination. Am J Surg 1971;122:74–7.

58. Hunt TK. Anaerobic metabolism and wound healing: a hypothesis for the initiation and cessation of collagen synthesis in wounds. Am J Surg 1978;138:238.

59. Carrico TJ, Mehrof AI, Cohen IK. Biology of wound healing. Surg Clin North Am 1984;64:721–33.

60. Douglas DM, Forrester JC, Ogilvie RR. Physical stages of collagen in later stages of wound healing. Br J Surg 1969;56:219–22.

61. Pickett BP, Burgess LP, Livermore GH, et al. Wound healing. Tensile strength vs healing time for wounds closed under tension. Arch Otolaryngol Head Neck Surg 1996;122:565–8.

62. Yamamoto LG. Preventing adverse events and outcomes encountered using Dermabond. Am J Emerg Med 2000;18:511–5.

63. Noordiz JP, Foresman PA, Rodeheaver GT, et al. Tissue adhesive wound repair revisited. J Emerg Med 1994;12:645–9.

64. Yaron M, Halperin M, Huffer W, Cairns C. Efficacy for tissue glue repair in an animal model. Acad Emerg Med 1995;2:259–63.

65. Saxena AK, Willital GH. Octylcyanoacrylate tissue adhesive in the repair of pediatric extremity lacerations. Am Surg 1999;65:470–2.

66. Steiner Z, Mogilner J. [Histoacryl vs Dermabond cyanoacrylate glue for closing small operative wounds]. Harefuah 2000;139:409–11, 496.

67. Edlich RF, Rodeheaver GT, Morgan RF, et al. Principles of emergency wound management. Ann Emerg Med 1988;17:1284–302.

68. Cardany CR, Rodheaver G, Edgerton MT, Edlich RF. The crush injury: a high risk wound. JACEP 1976;5:965–70.

69. Kligman AM. The bacteriology of normal skin. In: Maibach HI, Hildick-Smith, editors. Skin bacteria and their role in infection. McGraw Hill Book Company; 1965. p. 13–21.

70. Duncan WC, McBride ME, Knox JM. Experimental production for cutaneous bacterial infection in humans. J Invest Dermatol 1970;54:319–23.

71. Hollander JE, Singer AJ, Valentine S, et al. Wound registry: development and validation. Ann Emerg Med 1995;25:675–85.

72. Ellis GL. Detection of soft tissue foreign bodies by plain radiography, xerography, computerized axial tomography, and ultrasonography. Ann Emerg Med 1989;18:161.

73. Waldbillig DK, Quinn JV, Stiell IG, Wells GA. Randomized double blind controlled trial comparing room temperature and heated lidocaine for digital nerve block. Ann Emerg Med 1995;26:677–81.

74. Brogan GX, Giarrusso E, Hollander JE, et al. Comparison of plain, warmed, and buffered lidocaine for anesthesia of traumatic wounds. Ann Emerg Med 1995;26:121–5.

75. Schilling CG, Bank DE, Borchert BA, et al. Tetracaine, epinephrine (adrenaline), and cocaine (TAC) vs lidocaine, epinephrine, and tetracaine (LET) for anesthesia of lacerations in children. Ann Emerg Med 1995;25:203–8.

76. Powell DM, Rodeheaver GT, Foresman PA, et al. Damage to tissue defences by EMLA cream. J Emerg Med 1991;9:205.

77. Zempsky WT, Karasic RB. EMLA vs TAC for topical anesthesia of extremity wounds in children. Ann Emerg Med 1997;30:163–6.

78. Dailey RH. Fatality secondary to misuse of TAC solution. Ann Emerg Med 1988;17:159.

79. LET preparation. Am J Health-Syst Pharm 1996;53:659.

80. Seropian R, Reynolds BM. Wound infections after preoperative depilation versus razor preparation. Am J Surg 1971;121:251–4.

81. Faddis D, Daniel D, Boyer J. Tissue toxicity of antiseptic solutions. A study of rabbit articular and periartical tissues. J Trauma 1977;17:895–7.

82. Oberg MS, Lindsey D. Do not put hydrogen peroxide or povidone iodine into wounds. J Trauma 1980;20:323–4.

83. Hollander JE, Richman PB, Werblud M, et al. Irrigation in facial and scalp lacerations: does it alter outcome? Ann Emerg Med 1998;31:73–7.

84. Moscati R, Mayrose J, Fincher L, Jehle D. Comparison of normal saline with tap water for wound irrigation. Am J Emerg Med 1998;16:379–81.

85. Moscati RM, Reardon RF, Lerner EB, Mayrose J. Wound irrigation with tap water. Acad Emerg Med 1998;5:1076–80.

86. Bansal BC, Wiebe RA, Perkins SD, Abramo TJ. Tap water for irriga-

tion of lacerations. Am J Emerg Med 2002;20:469–72.

87. Dire DJ, Welsh AP. A comparison of wound irrigation solutions used in the emergency department. Ann Emerg Med 1990;19:704–8.

88. Singer AJ, Hollander JE, Subramanian S, et al. Pressure dynamics of various irrigation techniques commonly used in the emergency department. Ann Emerg Med 1994;24:36–40.

89. Wray CR. Force required for wound closue and scar appearance. Plast Reconstr Surg 1983;72:380–2.

90. Thacker JG, Iachetta FA, Allaire PE, et al. Biomechanical properties—their influence on planning surgical incisions. In: Krizek TJ, Hoops PE, editors. Symposium on basic science in plastic surgery. Vol 15. CV Mosby; 1975. p. 72–9.

91. Phillips LG, Heggers JP. Layered closure of lacerations. Postgrad Med 1988;83:142–8.

92. Traub AC QF. Cutaneous wound closure: early staple removal and replacement by skin tapes. Contemp Surg 1981;18.

93. Mehta PH, Dunn KA, Bradfield JF, Austin PE. Contaminated wounds: infection rates with subcutaneous sutures. Ann Emerg Med 1996;27:43–8.

94. Rouvelas H, Saffra N, Rosen M. Inadvertent tarsorrhaphy secondary to Dermabond. Pediatr Emerg Care 2000;16:346.

95. Leahy AB, Gottsch JD, Stark WJ. Clinical experience with n-butyl-cyanoacrylate (Nexacryl) tissue adhesive. Ophthalmology 1993;100:173–8.

96. Mertz PM, Davis SC, Cazzaniga AL, et al. Barrier and antibacterial properties of 2-octyl cyanoacrylate-derived wound treatment films. J Cutan Med Surg 2003;7:1–6.

97. Bhende S, Rothenburger S, Spangler DJ, Dito M. In vitro assessment of microbial barrier properties of Dermabond topical skin adhesive. Surg Infect (Larchmt) 2002;3:251–7.

98. Toriumi DM, O'Grady K, Desai D, Bagal A. Use of octyl-2-cyanoacrylate for skin closure in facial plastic surgery. Plast Reconstr Surg 1998;102:2209–19.

99. Osmond MH, Klassen TP, Quinn JV. Economic comparison of a tissue adhesive and suturing in the repair of pediatric facial lacerations. J Pediatr 1995;126:892–5.

100. Quinn J, Lowe L, Mertz M. The effect of a new tissue-adhesive wound dressing on the healing of traumatic abrasions. Dermatology 2000;201:343–6.

101. Singer A, Berrutti L, Thode HJ, McClain S. Octylcyanoacrylate for the treatment of partial-thickness burns in swine: a randomized, controlled experiment. Acad Emerg Med 1999;6:688–92.

102. Singer A, Berrutti L, McClain S. Comparative trial of octyl-cyanoacrylate and silver sulfadiazine for the treatment of full-thickness

skin wounds. Wound Repair Regen 1999;7:356–61.

103. Singer AJ, Mohammad M, Tortora G, et al. Octylcyanoacrylate for the treatment of contaminated partial-thickness burns in swine: a randomized controlled experiment. Acad Emerg Med 2000;7:222–7.

104. Singer A, Thode H Jr, McClain S. The effects of octylcyanoacrylate on scarring after burns. Acad Emerg Med 2001;8:107–11.

105. Singer AJ, Nable M, Cameau P, et al. Evaluation of a new liquid occlusive dressing for excisional wounds. Wound Repair Regen 2003;11:181–7.

106. Mertz PM, Davis SC, Cazzaniga AL, et al. Barrier and antibacterial properties of 2-octyl cyanoacrylate-derived wound treatment films. J Cutan Med Surg 2003;7:1–6.

107. n-Butyl cyanoacrylate embolization of cerebral arteriovenous malformations: results of a prospective, randomized, multi-center trial. AJNR Am J Neuroradiol 2002;23:748–55.

108. Suh DC, Kim KS, Lim SM, et al. Technical feasibility of embolizing aneurysms with glue (n-butyl 2-cyanoacrylate): experimental study in rabbits. AJNR Am J Neuroradiol 2003;24:1532–9.

4 Fibrin-Based Adhesives and Hemostatic Agents

WILLIAM D. SPOTNITZ, MD, SANDRA G. BURKS, BSN, ROSHAN PRABHU, BS

The craft of surgery has evolved over centuries. Suture-like threads created from a wide variety of substances were used as early as the second century BC for mechanical closure of wounds. The concept of using surgical glue, on the other hand, to approximate the skin edges of wounds or to cause adherence of other tissues is a relatively new idea.[1] In fact, the US Food and Drug Administration (FDA) approved the introduction of the first widely accepted tissue glue in 1998. This new glue, fibrin sealant, represents the first model for an industry that is rapidly evolving. There are now five new families of surgical adhesives and hemostats, including fibrin sealant, cyanoacrylate, bovine collagen and thrombin, polyethylene glycol polymer, and albumin cross-linked with glutaraldehyde.[2] The development of safe and efficacious agents is now beginning to satisfy an important surgical need that is increasing as more minimally invasive and technically challenging operations are being undertaken by surgeons. Just as the fine cabinetmaker has benefited from the use of saws, nails, and glues, so has the master surgeon benefited from well-designed scalpels, specialized sutures, and now surgical adhesives. The introduction of new surgical adhesives and hemostats will allow surgeons to perform operations using smaller and smaller incisions with less tissue trauma. Their use will decrease bleeding and improve outcomes. This should result in improved cost-effectiveness as well.

The ideal surgical tissue adhesive, however, has not yet been created and, in fact, may not be a reasonable expectation. For example, at present, surgeons employ a wide variety of different sutures. There are multiple types and sizes of sutures, including those that are absorbable or nonabsorbable. Surgeons from different specialties will also require different characteristics in a surgical tissue adhesive. In a perfect operative environment, the ideal tissue adhesive agent has several basic characteristics.

First, the ideal tissue adhesive needs to be "safe." Thus, there should be no danger with respect to the use of the agent or its breakdown products. There should be no risk of metabolic, infectious, immunologic, or oncologic complications. The material should not interfere with any metabolic pathways that would produce significant biologic dysfunction. There should be no risk of bacterial, viral, or other identified or unidentified infectious agents being transmitted as the result of the use of the agent. The adhesive should not have any significant antigenic capacity and should not provide danger to the patient on repetitive exposure. The adhesive and its metabolites should not be capable of producing a malignancy. Preferably, these materials should be completely biodegradable so that there will be no long-term effects as a result of their use. Second, the tissue adhesive should be highly "effective." This is a difficult requirement because effectiveness will vary with each specialty and each application. For example, a vascular surgeon creating an anastomosis between two segments of an artery may require an agent that is rapidly polymerizing and has some inherent hemostatic capacity. Thus, the material needs to be capable of preventing bleeding from the anastomosis by sealing any potential openings and needs to be capable of causing a site of active bleeding to clot without clotting the anastomosis itself. On the contrary, a cosmetic surgeon performing facial reconstruction may require an agent that polymerizes more slowly, allowing for the precise arrangement of flaps, grafts, and tissues prior to permanent fixation to produce the best cosmetic result. Thus, effectiveness may be different for each surgical specialist. Third, the material needs to be easily "usable." There are multiple aspects to this requirement. The ability to reconstitute the agent and prepare it for use in the operating room in a rapid and efficient manner is important. This is becoming even more relevant in an era of decreasing operating room personnel resources and continuing efforts to improve efficiency and cost-effectiveness. Products that can be stored easily and maintain their effectiveness with a prolonged shelf life are advantageous. Also, materials that can be prepared for application rapidly are desirable. In this setting, no advance notice is required from the surgeon to support staff, and the staff is not unduly preoccupied with preparation. Once the agent is prepared and available for the surgeon, the convenience and versatility of the applicators are also important. An applicator that allows the precise placement of the tissue adhesive to both specific localized areas and over more diffuse broad surfaces is desirable. For example, a pointed-tip applicator (Figure 4-1), which will allow placement of the tissue adhesive on a linear suture line, and a spray attachment, which will allow distribution of a thin layer of material over a larger surface area, are required. Not only are different types of applicator tips important, but also the length of the applicator needs to be variable. A general surgeon may require a long, narrow applicator capable of use through a laparoscope, whereas an ophthalmologist may require a shorter, finer device capable of extremely precise and controlled delivery. Fourth, the adhesive needs to be "affordable." The hospital administrator and pharmacist's decision to stock the material and the surgeon's decision to use the agent in the operating room are influenced significantly by the cost-effectiveness of the product. Unfortunately, there is a relative lack of cost-effectiveness data with respect to the use of surgical adhesives and hemostats. Clinical trials demonstrating that the use of these materials, including the expense of the agents themselves, results in a decrease in overall costs associated with a specific procedure would be very useful. Such data would not only justify the clinical value of the agent but also would support its use in an increasingly cost-conscious environment. Fifth and finally, the product needs to be "approvable." Although this seems inherently obvious at first

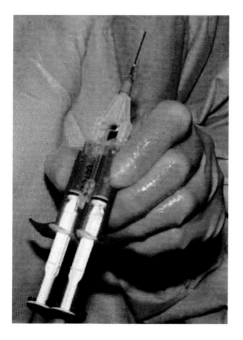

■ FIGURE 4–1   System for linear application of fibrin sealant using a needle-tipped applicator.

glance, this issue has been critical in the development of tissue adhesives in the United States. Fibrin sealant was commercially available in Europe for a quarter of a century before it was finally approved for use by the FDA in 1998. Thus, demonstrations of safety and clinically relevant and scientifically significant efficacy were not initially straightforward in the emerging field of tissue adhesives. Recent modifications of FDA guidelines for these materials are now allowing more effective, rapid, and efficient regulatory approval of these agents. Since 1998, multiple different individual agents and families of materials have now been approved. Second-generation products and entirely new materials are in various stages of the development and regulatory approval process.

Surgeons are inquisitive and capable physicians as well as craftsmen. They are willing to incorporate new products and devices into their operative armamentarium. However, the successful use of new tissue adhesives by fully trained practicing surgeons differs from the introduction of new medications. It requires a directed and specific educational effort. The use of these agents is also associated with a learning curve for the surgeon. Educational resources, including pamphlets, books, lectures, computer simulations, and hands-on laboratory experience, are valuable adjuncts for surgeons already in practice. Surgical residents in the process of acquiring and developing their technical skills will now be introduced to tissue adhesives as an additional element in their training. These individuals will be educated to use these agents for the proper indications in a safe and efficacious manner.

HISTORY

The history of fibrin sealant has been previously described.[3] Its use as a hemostat was described by Bergel in 1909.[4] In 1915, Lippencott described the use of fibrin for hemostatic purposes during cerebral surgery.[5] In 1940, Young and Medawar described the use of fibrinogen as an adhesive to achieve peripheral nerve attachment.[6] Cronkite and colleagues provided the first description of using both fibrinogen and thrombin as a biologic glue for the purposes of skin grafting in 1944.[7] The use of a fibrin sealant containing concentrated fibrinogen was described for neural anastomoses in 1982 by Matras and colleagues.[8] In the 1980s, Gestring and Lerner, Siedentop and colleagues, and Spotnitz and colleagues described clinically useful chemical and cryoprecipitation methods for producing concentrated fibrinogen for use in fibrin sealants.[9–11] Although fibrin sealant would not be approved as a commercial product for use in the United States for more than another 10 years, the material was being employed in this country using predominantly blood bank sources of fibrinogen, such as cryoprecipitate, or otherwise concentrated fibrinogen in combination with topical bovine thrombin. Experience in a wide variety of surgical specialties was documented in Europe using the commercial product[12] and in the United States using blood bank–derived fibrinogen.[13,14] The pivotal trial that was used in the regulatory process for approval of fibrin sealant by the FDA appeared in the literature in 1989.[15] Subsequent regulatory review based on safety and effectiveness data allowed approval of fibrin sealant as a commercial product in 1998. This has opened the modern era of tissue adhesive development and use in the United States and will lead to the addition of multiple, new, clinically useful products into the armamentarium of the American surgeon.

BIOCHEMISTRY AND TOXICITY

Fibrin sealant is formed from concentrated fibrinogen and thrombin. This biochemical reaction has been well delineated[16] and remains the subject of further study (Figure 4-2).[17] Fibrinogen molecules with the molecular weight of 340,000 Da and an elongated 45 nm structure

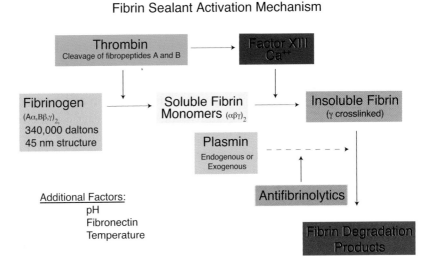

Fibrin Sealant Activation Mechanism

■ FIGURE 4–2 Diagram of the mechanism of action of fibrin sealant.

are composed of two sets of polypeptide chains, $(A_\alpha, B_\beta, \gamma)_2$. In the presence of thrombin, the fibrin of peptides, A and B, is cleaved, leading to the formation of soluble fibrin monomers ($\alpha\beta\gamma$) that form twisting fibrils and fibers of a three-dimensional network. In the presence of factor XIII and calcium as catalysts, γ cross-linking occurs to form the insoluble fibrin that is the final form of fibrin sealant. Additional factors that can influence the formation of this material include pH, fibronectin, and temperature. The final fibrin sealant is subject to fibrinolytic degradation by both endogenous and exogenous plasmin. Antifibrinolytics such as aprotinin, tranexamic acid, and ε-aminocaproic acid can be added to the mixture to reduce the rate of fibrinolysis and creation of fibrin degradation products.[18]

The safety concerns associated with the use of fibrin sealant are predominantly related to the risk of disease transmission or the negative effects of the antifibrinolytics used in these agents. Specifically, the risk of viral disease transmission exists as a result of the pooled human plasma that is used to create the concentrated fibrinogen and thrombin required for this two-component sealant. The commercial manufacturers of fibrin sealant make extensive efforts to reduce the risk of viral disease transmission. The antifibrinolytics used in the presently produced material also have some associated immunologic or biochemical risks.

The first commercial product approved in 1998, Tisseel, distributed in the United States by Baxter Healthcare Corp. (Glendale, CA), uses cryoprecipitation and freeze-drying to eliminate viruses from both the fibrinogen and the thrombin components. It also uses Sephadex (cross-linked dextran beads) adsorption to further reduce the risk of viral transmission in the thrombin component. Reported log inactivation numbers for this commercial product are greater than 5.6 to 7.[19] This product contains aprotinin as an antifibrinolytic agent of bovine origin. There are reports of allergic reactions to this protein. These may vary from skin rash to anaphylaxis and death.[20,21] The risk of hypersensitivity reaction caused by immunoglobulin E antibodies against bovine aprotinin is reported to be rare in patients without prior exposure but may be as high as 5% between 2 weeks and 6 months after the first exposure.[22]

In 2003, the American Red Cross entered the fibrin sealant market with a second-generation fibrin sealant, Crosseal. This fibrin sealant product has additional antiviral processing in the form of solvent detergent cleansing with Triton X-100 for both fibrinogen and thrombin components and heat pasteurization for fibrinogen and nanofiltration for thrombin. The reported rates of viral inactivation for these processes are greater than 9.8 to 10.6 logs.[23] Crosseal contains synthetic tranexamic acid as an antifibrinolytic.[21] Although the use of tranexamic acid eliminates the risk of immunogenic reactions associated with aprotinin, its use in the central nervous system has been reported to cause hyperexcitability, convulsions, and death as a result of a $_\gamma$-aminobutyric acid receptor antagonism in animal models.[24–27] Thus, Crosseal is specifically contraindicated for applications in which it may come in contact with cerebrospinal fluid or dura mater.

Both of the presently available pooled plasma commercial products, Tisseel and Crosseal, could be associated with the transmission of unidentified viral or prion diseases, including those potentially causing Creutzfeldt-Jakob disease. There is no evidence that fibrin sealant is carcinogenic. It is biodegradable, so the long-term effects of the agent itself and its metabolites are minimal. There are no recent reports of significant fibrosis or tissue reaction using these materials.

Prior to the introduction of commercial products, concentrated fibrinogen obtained in the blood bank or by chemical precipitation was used in combination with topical bovine thrombin to produce fibrin sealant.[28,29] The bovine thrombin used with these forms of fibrinogen to produce fibrin sealant has been reported to cause antibody formation against human thrombin and factor V, potentially causing coagulopathy.[30,31]

Overall, fibrin sealant has a relatively good biocompatibility profile. It is fibrinolyzed over a period of weeks; thus, the risks from the agent, such as long-term fibrosis or carcinogenicity, are minimized.

CLINICAL USES, REGULATIONS, COSTS, AND EFFECTIVENESS

Fibrin sealant has been used in a wide variety of clinical applications. There are specific on-label indications for use of commercial fibrin sealants. There is also extensive literature supporting the use of fibrin sealant in a wide variety of off-label applications.

The commercial agents that are presently available for use in the United States are approved for hemostasis in operations involving cardiopulmonary bypass, splenic trauma, and liver resection, as well as sealing of colonic anastomoses at the time of colostomy closure. Thus, the on-label indications for fibrin sealant are basically hemostasis in cardiac, liver, and splenic procedures and sealing colonic anastomoses. In the following sections, the uses of fibrin sealant in a wide variety of surgical specialties are discussed. This discussion includes the on-label indications of hemostasis and sealing and the off-label uses, including drug delivery and tissue engineering.

Cardiac Surgery

Because cardiac surgery (Figure 4–3) involves major procedures frequently with multiple suture lines and requires the use of the cardiopulmonary bypass pump and heparin, it is subject to bleeding complications. Coagulopathy is established in these operations as a result of fibrinolysis and platelet dysfunction from the cardiopulmonary bypass pump and the use of heparin to prevent clotting in the bypass circuit. Although protamine is used at the end of these cases to reverse the effect of heparin and stop bleeding, agents that can enhance hemostasis during the operation are still particularly useful in this specialty. A randomized perspective clinical trial used to obtain fibrin sealant registration in the United States showed that this agent could be successfully used in cardiac surgical operations.[15] It reduced the volume of bleeding and need for reoperation in the patients who had this material employed during their procedures. There are extensive stud-

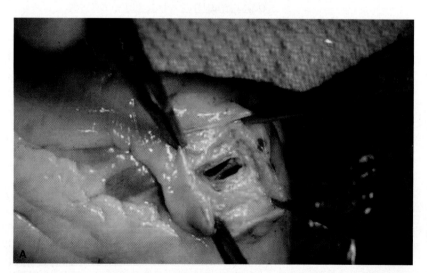

■ FIGURE 4–3   (A) Left ventriculotomy for excision of an apical clot. (B) Polytetrafluoroethylene (PTFE) patch for closure of a left ventriculotomy. (C) Closure of left ventricular muscle over a PTFE patch. (D) Layer of fibrin sealant sprayed on a left ventricular muscle closure.

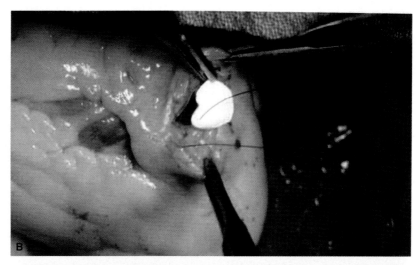

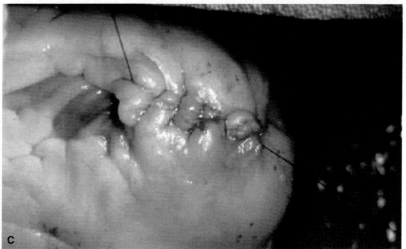

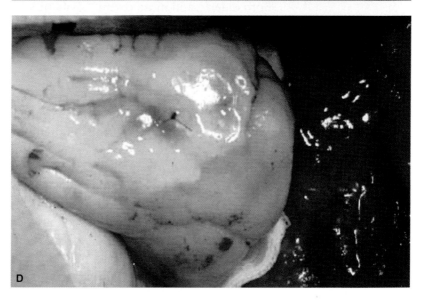

ies in the literature documenting the value of fibrin sealant in a wide variety of cardiac surgical applications.[13,32,33] The sealant can be used effectively as a hemostatic agent to stop bleeding from adhesions at the time of reoperative cardiac surgery and from diffuse surfaces with capillary bleeding. The agent is not a substitute for surgical sutures and excellent technique. It will not stop active arterial bleeding when a suture is required. Fibrin sealant can be applied through a pointed-tip applicator or as a spray. The pointed-tip applicator is appropriate for suture lines at large vessel anastomoses and is useful in both adult and pediatric cardiac surgical procedures. It is best used to seal anastomoses prior to pressurizing blood vessels. A polymerization time of 1 to 2 minutes should be used if possible prior to reestablishing pressurized blood flow. This allows the fibrin sealant to fully form and adhere prior to undergoing vascular pressure. At sites with active bleeding in which the liquid fibrin sealant may be washed away in advance of its polymerization, it is possible to deliver the fibrin sealant with a carrier sponge of cellulose or collagen, which will enhance the ability of the fibrin sealant to achieve hemostasis. There is a dramatic example of this method with the report of repair of a free wall rupture of the left ventricle using a fibrin sealant patch.[34]

In the European literature, a study recently supported the use of a patient-derived fibrin sealant that produces a fibrin I sealant capable of polymerizing in an alkaline environment and not requiring thrombin.[35,36] This agent is entirely autologous and depends on a bedside mechanical apparatus capable of deriving the fibrin I monomer from the patient's own blood.

Both older[15] and more recent[37] randomized, controlled studies support the use of fibrin sealant in cardiac surgical operations.[33]

Thoracic Surgery

The use of fibrin sealant in pulmonary resections remains controversial. This is an extremely difficult environment for surgical adhesives. Sealing the parenchyma of the lung requires a material that is both elastic and strongly adherent to the parenchymal surface. For the sealant to be properly applied, air leaks from the parenchymal surface must be absent during application, and this requires a relatively deflated lung. After application of the sealant has been completed, inflation of the lung can be resumed, but the parenchyma undergoes a significant surface area change. If the sealant is relatively inelastic and nonadherent, it will easily snap off from the surface of the lung during this period of surface area transformation. If, on the other hand, the sealant is highly elastic and strongly adherent, it will remain attached to the parenchymal surface, stretch, and serve as an excellent means of achieving pneumostasis. There are reports in the literature in support of the use of fibrin sealant not only for sealing parenchymal air leaks but also for closing those of the bronchial tree.[38] However, controversy exists. An article suggesting a lack of effect of fibrin sealant[39] directly applied to the lung and an article supporting a significant benefit[40] of fibrin sealant sprayed on the lung parenchyma have appeared in the recent literature. Efforts to increase the strength of fibrin sealant to allow for more effective use by combining it with collagen have been described.[41] Successful use of fibrin sealant to stop persistent parenchymal air leaks using the thoracoscope[42] and the bronchoscope for bronchopleural fistulae[43,44] has been reported.

Vascular Surgery

Fibrin sealant is an effective means of sealing vascular anastomoses prior to pressurizing blood vessels at the time of vascular clamp removal (Figure 4–4). Thus, the anastomoses can be reinforced with fibrin sealant prior to the return of circulation, allowing the sealant to polymerize for a period of at least 1 to 2 minutes before repressurization. This is an excellent way of achieving hemostasis and has been shown to be superior to presently available techniques, including manual pressure, bovine thrombin, and oxidized regenerated cellulose to achieve hemostasis in polypropylene sewn anastomoses performed with polytetrafluoroethylene (PTFE) grafts.[45,46] In the laboratory, a variety of different techniques have been employed to allow the use of fibrin sealant to support anastomoses performed with a reduced number of sutures[47] or even no sutures.[48,49]

A word of caution needs to be given when using tissue adhesives with microvascular anastomoses. In particular, fibrin sealant with concentrations of thrombin in excess of 500 IU/mL may contribute to an increased rate of thrombosis in venous anastomoses.[50,51]

Finally, it should be noted that a significant body of literature supports the use of fibrin sealant as a drug delivery system for medications capable of reducing endothelial hyperplasia associated with vascular grafts at surgical anastomoses.[52] It can also be used as a method of attaching endothelial cells to artificial grafts to create a new endothelial lining.[53] Fibrin sealant has been reported to be a satisfactory means of providing external support to vein grafts that will be subjected to arterial pressures. In this setting, it appears to reduce endothelial cell injury.[54]

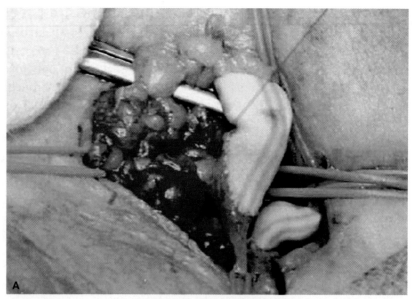

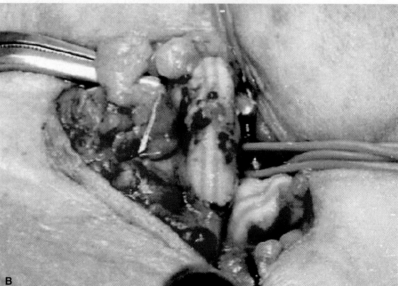

■ FIGURE 4–4   (A) Completed anastomosis after placement of a poly-tetrafluoroethylene shunt for hemodialysis. (B) Fibrin sealant on anastomosis to ensure hemostasis from needle holes following polypropylene suturing.

Oncologic Surgery

The use of fibrin sealant in operations for the treatment of tumors is primarily restricted to elimination of postresection seromas and fluid accumulations and the experimental, local delivery of chemotherapeutic agents.

With respect to the prevention of seromas, fibrin sealant has been shown in both animal and human models to be an effective method for causing adherence of the skin to underlying muscle after resection of breast or axillary tissue to prevent fluid accumulation. This method eliminates the potential space and also seals lymphatics and capillaries.[55–59] However, this area is associated with disagreement. Several authors have found fibrin sealant to be ineffective in reducing seroma formation and wound drainage at the time of mastectomy and axillary dissection.[60,61] The explanation for this discrepancy may be related to methods of application. If fibrin sealant is applied between two surfaces and these surfaces are brought in immediate contact while the adhesive is polymerizing, then an effective bond is formed. This bond eliminates the potential space and seals any capillaries or lymphatics within the space. However, if the fibrin sealant is applied to one surface and a delay occurs between apposition of the two surfaces to be bonded together, then the material paradoxically functions as an excellent antiadhesive. In other words, if polymerization is completed with the two surfaces not in contact and they then come together after completion of polymerization, the smooth layer of fibrin sealant effectively prevents adhesion between the two surfaces. This delay of apposition may actually create a seroma of a larger magnitude than might have occurred if no fibrin sealant had been used. The best method of wound closure to prevent this problem and to allow for immediate contact of the skin and underlying muscle is to place a latticework of suture prior to applying the fibrin sealant.[56] After application of the fibrin sealant, the latticework is immediately pulled tight, and the skin comes in contact with the underlying muscle. This contact is facilitated by direct manual pressure application onto the skin for a period of 1 to 2 minutes. In this setting, polymerization of the fibrin sealant occurs with the two layers in contact. They become adherent. Because the skin closure has been preplaced, there is no necessity to further move the skin. No disruption of the underlying bonds between the skin and muscle as a result of suture placement will occur. This is also an important concept because any pulling up on the skin with a forceps to place additional sutures can disrupt the fibrin sealant bond between the skin and muscle. If this bond is disrupted, there is again the situation in which an excellent antiadhesive lies between the skin and muscle. This antiadhesive may predispose the patient to excessive serous drainage. The proper understanding and use of fibrin sealant are important in this setting and will allow for the appropriate use of fibrin sealant as either an adhesive or an antiadhesive in a wide variety of specialties.

Fibrin sealant can also be used as a drug delivery system for a variety of different medications. Specifically, it is capable of local drug release of chemotherapeutic agents. This occurs by two mechanisms.

First, there is direct diffusion of molecules from the fibrin sealant. Larger molecules diffuse out of the material at a slower rate, whereas smaller molecules diffuse out more rapidly. Second, there is fibrinolysis, producing a breakdown of the fibrin sealant, which causes release of the drug as well. This rate can be regulated by the concentration of antifibrinolytic agent within the fibrin sealant. Thus, fibrin sealant may be an effective delivery system for chemotherapeutic agents to solid and bony tumors.[62–64]

Plastic Surgery

There are three major applications of fibrin sealant in plastic surgery.[65] First, it can be used effectively as a hemostatic agent following burn débridement with or without skin grafting. Second, the fibrin sealant can also be used to immediately attach the new graft and improve graft survival in a variety of different clinical situations. Also, as was mentioned earlier, the material is capable of reducing the need for drains in a wide variety of procedures, including muscle flaps and extensive soft tissue dissections. In facial and cosmetic surgery, fibrin sealant has been particularly useful in reducing and facilitating endoscopic procedures.[66] The benefits of fibrin sealants in assisting with burn wound treatment and skin graft placement have been well summarized.[67] Not only can the fibrin sealant help with achieving hemostasis by causing coagulation at the sites of burn wound débridement, but it can also help with successful placement of the skin grafts themselves. Even in difficult to reach normally inaccessible sites, the use of fibrin sealant may help in the attachment and survival or "take" of a skin graft. The product may eliminate the need for bolus dressings, sutures, or clips to assist with the fixation of the graft. It is important to remember that only a thin layer of fibrin sealant should be used in this setting.[68] The surgeon needs to avoid an excessively thick adhesion barrier between the graft itself and the underlying tissue that could contribute to a decrease in graft "take." Third and finally, it has been documented in patients undergoing facelift that drains can be successfully eliminated.[69] It is reported that significant reductions in hematoma formation, edema, and ecchymosis can be achieved by the use of fibrin sealant.

Neurosurgery

Fibrin sealant is particularly useful in neurosurgical procedures. Operations on the central nervous system can result in cerebrospinal fluid leakage, which can persist as a permanent leak. There is no inherent clotting ability in the cerebrospinal fluid. Thus, a watertight seal on all central nervous system suture lines is critically important and can be facilitated using fibrin sealant. The agent has been documented to be helpful both in prophylactic treatment and in treatment to eliminate established cerebrospinal fluid fistulae.[70] These fistulae can be treated with subcutaneous application of fibrin sealant as well.[71]

Fibrin sealant has been demonstrated to be effective in repairing frontal sinuses using free autologous bone grafts obtained at the time of craniotomy.[72] This reduces the risks of complications that are associated with more traditional techniques, including vascularized periosteum, gallia, or resected fatty tissue and muscle. However, it is worth remembering that there has been at least one report of a spinal arachnoid cyst at the time of closure of a suboccipital bone defect. This could potentially have been related to fibrin sealant application. It was speculated that the fibrin sealant used might have blocked cerebrospinal fluid drainage, leading to cyst formation.[73]

Finally, fibrin sealant has been used in neurosurgical procedures to reattach peripheral nerves. The material may reduce inflammation associated with sutures and enhance axonal regeneration. Most of this nerve attachment work has been performed in the experimental laboratory and still remains controversial. The use of fibrin sealant for nerve attachment has not gained widespread clinical acceptance.

Ophthalmologic Surgery

Fibrin sealant has been employed successfully during ophthalmologic procedures to close conjunctival wounds with less discomfort than sutures.[74] It has also been used to close corneal perforations and deep ulcers.[75] In this setting, it has been noted to produce faster healing and less vascularization than treatment with cyanoacrylate.

Orthopedic Surgery

Joint replacement surgery in orthopedics can be associated with significant blood loss. Early anticoagulation of these patients is, however, desirable in an effort to prevent deep venous thrombosis and the life-threatening complication of pulmonary embolus. Thus, these operations are settings in which fibrin sealant may be useful. The literature supports significant reductions in blood loss using fibrin sealant in both knee replacement[76-78] (Figure 4–5) and hip replacement.[79]

Fibrin sealant has also been effective in orthopedic surgery to increase ingrowth during repair of tendons and articular defects, enhance bone induction, improve bone graft filling, strengthen fracture fixation, facilitate spinal fusion, and assist with implant fixation.[14]

Trauma Surgery

This product has been successfully used as an adjunct to solid organ injury in patients sustaining severe abdominal trauma.[80] In fact, the commercial fibrin sealants on the market in the United States, Crosseal and Tisseel, have been approved for use in liver and splenic surgery, respectively. Thus, these agents are useful in reducing bleeding in the parenchyma of the liver and spleen. This is a particularly useful application in liver procedures that can be associated with significant blood loss and the need for transfusions. Spleens, on the other hand, can be removed rapidly to avoid blood loss, but significant clinical evidence supports splenic salvage as opposed to splenectomy as the best treatment for patients. This is because splenic repair allows patients to maintain their immune responses to encapsulated organisms, particularly pneumococcus. Thus, fibrin sealant can be a valuable adjunct to both liver and spleen procedures. The development of fibrin sealant dressings or bandages for use with massive extremity wounds and other soft tissue injuries applicable to mass causality situations is also under way, although no commercial products are presently approved for use by the FDA in the United States.[81,82]

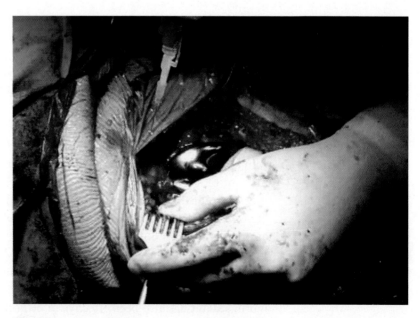

■ FIGURE 4–5   Application of fibrin sealant during total knee arthroplasty.

Head and Neck Surgery

This specialty has used fibrin sealant as a mucosal barrier, a method of seroma prevention (Figure 4–6), a substitute for nonabsorbable packing, and a carrier for bone fillers. There is evidence to support the use of fibrin sealant as a mucosal barrier at the time of tonsillectomy as a means of reducing bleeding and pain following these procedures.[83,84] It has been used to eliminate the use of drains for removal of serous fluid and can potentially reduce the risk of salivary fistula formation at the time of parotidectomy.[85] Fibrin sealant has been used to eliminate the need for packing at the time of endoscopic sinus surgery and has improved patient comfort while reducing the risks of complications.[86,87] The use of fibrin sealant combined with bone filler, such as hydroxyapatite granules and calcium phosphate, has been described in the treatment of atrophic rhinitis.[88] A literature review of fibrin sealant in otologic and neurotologic procedures does warn against the use of an excessive amount of fibrin sealant applied in a thick manner.[89] Application in this way can impair healing and potentially predispose the patient to pseudopolyps, granulomas, and fibromas. Recent publications suggest that fibrin sealant is capable of reducing complications at the time of nasal septal procedures.[90]

Gynecologic and Urologic Surgery

In gynecologic procedures, fibrin sealant has been used to enhance embryo transfer by improving adherence at the time of in vitro fertilization.[91] Both gynecologists and neurologists have used it to help with endoscopic[92] and transvaginal colposuspension.[93] Fibrin sealant has been used successfully on multiple occasions to seal premature rupture of amniotic membrane.[94–97]

With respect to urologic surgery, fibrin sealant is gaining increased use for a wide variety of applications.[98,99] These include animal studies supporting its use for microsurgical anastomosis, fistula repair, circumcision, laparoscopy, and tissue engineering. A recent report supports its use in genital and urinary injuries, fistulae, and urologic surgical complications.[100]

Gastrointestinal Surgery

The use of fibrin sealant for sealing gastrointestinal anastomoses, particularly for colonic anastomosis, remains controversial, with the literature reporting mixed results.[101–104] Several of these articles attempt to use fibrin sealant in extremely challenging situations,

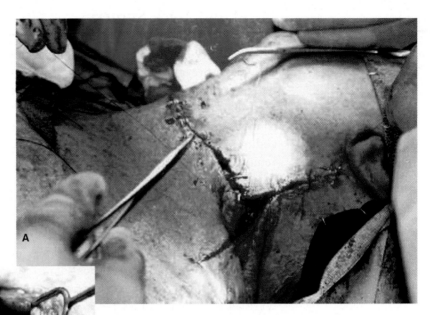

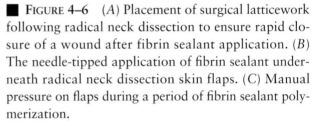

■ FIGURE 4–6 (A) Placement of surgical latticework following radical neck dissection to ensure rapid closure of a wound after fibrin sealant application. (B) The needle-tipped application of fibrin sealant underneath radical neck dissection skin flaps. (C) Manual pressure on flaps during a period of fibrin sealant polymerization.

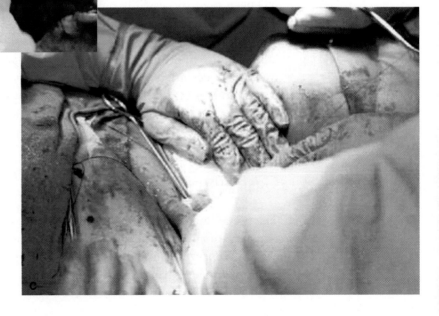

including fecal peritonitis and high-risk sutured anastomoses. However, commercial fibrin sealant has been approved by the FDA as an adjunct to colonic anastomoses at the time of colostomy closure.[19]

This product has been advocated in the laparoscopic treatment of perforated peptic ulcers with a fibrin sealant patch method superior to a sutured patch technique in terms of surgical performance.[105] Recent literature using fibrin sealant for bleeding gastric varices suggests mixed results, with some articles supporting its use[106,107] and others suggesting that it may carry a significant risk of rebleeding.[108] With respect to endoscopic treatment of bleeding peptic ulcers, using fibrin sealant in addition to epinephrine or instead of epinephrine has also met with mixed results, with no obvious significant improvement in clinical outcomes.[109,110]

Over the last 5 years, a large body of literature has developed on the use of fibrin sealant for anal fistulae. More than 14 clinical studies have been performed. The majority of reports support its use because it is easier, less painful, and less likely to cause anal incontinence. The method is associated with an intermediate chance of success. The literature supports its use as a less invasive and conservative approach and suggests that its success rates can be improved by using endoscopy, fluoroscopy, and repeated treatments, particularly in patients with complex anal fistulae.[111–114] Articles opposing its use suggest that its long-term success rate may be small. Magnetic resonance imaging long-term evaluation for patients with complex anal fistulae suggests a fibrin sealant success rate as low as 15%.[115,116]

A wide variety of other abdominal fistulae have been closed using fibrin sealant.[14]

Dental Surgery

The literature suggests an advantage to using fibrin sealant at the time of dental extractions in combination with tranexamic acid mouthwash and sutures. It appears to reduce bleeding at the time of dental extractions in patients with coagulopathies from hemophilia or therapeutic anticoagulation with warfarin.[117,118] A more recent animal study suggests that fibrin sealant used to fill extracted molar cavities results in less foreign-body reaction, abscess formation, and necrosis.[119] Controversy still exists with respect to the use of fibrin sealant for a gingival recession, with some authors favoring it[120] and others noting no improvement with its use.[121,122]

Drug Delivery and Tissue Engineering

Fibrin sealant as a result of its drug delivery capacity and biologic structure can serve as an effective mechanism for delivering a variety of different medications and a structural scaffold for tissue engineering. With respect to drug delivery, fibrin sealant has been demonstrated to be an excellent mechanism for delivery of antibiotics,[123] growth factors,[124] chemotherapeutic agents,[63] and topical anesthetics.[125] In addition, the literature supports the use of fibrin sealant with antibiotics to reduce postoperative ocular infections,[126] to treat localized peritoneal infections,[127] and to treat osteomyelitis.[128] Recent contributions to the fibrin sealant growth factor delivery literature suggest a positive effect on nerve regeneration.[129,130]

Fibrin sealant can also be used as a scaffold for cellular attachment and growth in the field of tissue engineering. It is capable of attaching cells and can provide a supportive environment for cellular growth and differentiation. Recent contributions to this literature include the use of fibrin sealant to assist with the construction of skin,[131–133] cartilage,[134] and bone.[135]

APPLICATION TECHNIQUES

There are a wide variety of clinical applications for fibrin sealant. The major categories include reduced hemorrhage, increased tissue plane adherence, drug delivery, and tissue engineering. The literature on these topics is extensive. It is beyond the scope of this chapter to review all of this information in depth. The above sections under clinical uses have presented many of the most recent human and animal studies in these four areas.

In this section, suggestions for the best and most effective clinical application of fibrin sealant are provided.

Available Products

Tisseel was approved in June 1998 for hemostasis at the time of operations involving cardiopulmonary bypass or splenic injury. It was also approved for an adjunct to colonic anastomosis at the time of colonostomy closure. This product contains pooled human fibrinogen and thrombin as well as bovine aprotinin. The product is virally inactivated using cryoprecipitation, freeze-drying, and vapor heating.

The thrombin component also undergoes adsorption. This product requires storage at 2 to 6°C as lyophilized powders that are reconstituted with saline in a thawing and mixing process that takes approximately 20 minutes of preparation time. The manufacturer provides multiple application devices, including needle, spray, and endoscopic tips. The cost is approximately $100 per 1 mL kit.

A second-generation fibrin sealant, Crosseal, was approved for commercial sale in March 2003. A license has been provided for using this product as a hemostatic agent at the time of liver resection surgery. The product contains pooled human fibrinogen and thrombin, as well as synthetic tranexamic acid. Antiviral processing includes cryoprecipitation and solvent detergent cleansing, as well as additional pasteurization of the fibrinogen component and immunofiltration of the thrombin component. The product is provided in liquid form that is stored at –18°C or colder. The frozen liquids can be thawed in a 2 to 8°C refrigerator within a day or at room temperature (20–25°C) within a period of 1 hour. Once thawed, the vials can be stored for rapid use in a refrigerator at 2 to 8°C for up to 30 days. Assembly of the product into an applicator is done with a needleless system. The applicator itself comes with various-length flexible tips that have a triple lumen that prevents clotting and clogging. It allows for linear application or aerosolized spray application. The cost is $100 to $150 for a 1 mL kit.

A third commercial system for producing fibrin sealant, CoStasis (Cohesion Technologies, US Surgical), combines bovine collagen and bovine thrombin with autologous plasma obtained in a centrifugation process from the patient. This product was approved in June 2000 as a device to stop active surgical bleeding during general surgical, hepatic, orthopedic, and cardiovascular procedures. The preparation time is that which is required to obtain autologous blood from the patient, perform the centrifugation steps that allow for preparation of plasma, and combine the plasma with bovine thrombin and collagen in the applicator device. The cost is approximately $100 to $150 for a 1 mL kit.

A variety of noncommercial methods for producing concentrated fibrinogen for combination with commercial bovine thrombin to produce fibrin sealant exist, including cryoprecipitation[11] and chemical precipitation.[10] Newer devices capable of producing the components required for fibrin sealant from the patient's own blood exist[136] and have reached commercialization in Europe. A computerized system capable of cryoprecipitating human fibrinogen in less than 1 hour

(CryoSeal AHS, Thermogenesis, Sacramento, CA) is also available and produces a fibrinogen concentration of approximately 27 mg/mL.[137] Methods of obtaining fibrinogen and thrombin using genetic engineering technologies in animals are under development.

Applications

In this section, a detailed discussion of the best methods of clinically employing fibrin sealant for successful use in several areas is provided. Specifically, the technique of using fibrin sealant to reduce bleeding, create successful vascular anastomoses, ensure satisfactory tissue apposition, achieve pneumostasis at the time of lung resection, and reduce lymphatic drainage by achieving lymphostasis is discussed.

With respect to bleeding, it must be said that the use of fibrin sealant is not a substitute for excellent surgical technique. If a surgical suture is required to control hemorrhage, it is best to use this technique as opposed to using fibrin sealant. However, for nonsuturable hemorrhage, fibrin sealant provides an excellent modality that should be included in every surgeon's armamentarium. Fibrin sealant is best applied to a dry field. Drying the area with a sponge and using the gas-driven spray applicator are effective methods to create a dry field. The use of gas from the applicator to remove blood prior to adding the two-component fibrin sealant mixture is an excellent technique of rapidly achieving a dry field. Thus, prior to applying the aerosolized fibrin sealant, the gas flow alone can be used to remove blood or other liquids from the operative field. The spray technique is particularly valuable for diffuse areas of capillary bleeding often encountered at the time of reoperative surgical dissections or when diffuse capillary or venous bleeding is encountered from inflamed tissues. The spray technique is particularly useful to cover large surface areas of bleeding. It also results in the most efficient use of the fibrin sealant, thus reducing the costs associated with the use of the agent.

If a localized area of bleeding is encountered, it may be best to use the needle or tip applicators provided by the manufacturer for specific application of the fibrin sealant at a small site. Some applicators are single lumen and may need to be changed if a period of delay occurs between fibrin sealant applications because these tips may become clogged. The manufacturer provides additional tips for these purposes, and some tip applicators are designed with multiple lumens to reduce the risk of clogging. Such point application with a tip applicator can be useful for sealing anastomosis in a wide variety of surgical procedures.

It should be noted that as presently commercially available, fibrin sealant is a two-component liquid adhesive. Thus, an active stream of bleeding will wash away the fibrin sealant prior to the 30 seconds required for initial polymerization. The application of fibrin sealant to an actively bleeding muscle or tissue is difficult, particularly for arterial bleeding. The best approach for using fibrin sealant in this situation is to combine it with a carrier sponge of cellulose or collagen. The fibrinogen component of the sealant can be applied to the sponge and allowed to soak into its interstices. Prior to applying the sponge to the actively bleeding area, the side of the sponge that will be applied directly to the bleeding site is activated with the thrombin component. Application of the components to the sponge can be done with a tipped or spray applicator. After activating the fibrinogen with the thrombin component, the sponge is immediately brought in contact with the active bleeding site, applying the activated side directly to the desired location. Pressure is maintained for a period of 2 to 3 minutes while polymerization of the fibrin sealant progresses. If active bleeding can be stopped during this period of pressure application, hemostasis will be achieved in the majority of situations after pressure application to the sponge is completed. Obviously, however, if bleeding continues while pressure is being applied with the sponge at the site of active bleeding, when the period of 2 to 3 minutes of pressure application is finished, there will still be bleeding. Therefore, one can get an immediate indication of the likelihood of the success of the fibrin sealant application. If bleeding does not cease on applying the sponge immediately with pressure, then the bleeding will not be successfully stopped with this technique. The carrier sponge technique is also useful for bleeding from the parenchyma of visceral organs, such as the liver and the spleen. It can also be useful in well-defined spaces that automatically create pressure application on the sponge, such as the pericardium.

Fibrin sealant is an excellent agent to use for sealing vascular anastomoses. It can be useful in both arterial and venous blood vessels. It is best used prior to systemic pressurization of the anastomosis prior to release of vascular occlusion clamps. Thus, the fibrin sealant should be applied after sewing the anastomosis but prior to resuming systemic pressure. The entire anastomosis is coated with fibrin sealant liquid either through the tip applicator or the spray application device. A period of 2 minutes of anealing time is then used to allow for sufficient polymerization of the fibrin sealant to be completed. The vascular clamps can then be released, and needle holes and other small sites of bleeding will be well controlled. Fibrin sealant, similarly, is an effective way of sealing patches or anastomoses sewn between PTFE and native blood vessels. It is especially effective in sealing the needle holes associated with the use of polypropylene suture and PTFE grafts or patches. Thus, use of fibrin sealant prophylactically on fragile blood vessels or PTFE anastomoses can be considered. This is the most effective way of employing the agent prior to the establishment of active bleeding. If active hemorrhage is encountered at a vascular anastomosis, the most effective way of achieving hemostasis with fibrin sealant is the use of a carrier sponge as discussed above. This allows the fibrin sealant to be combined with pressure and avoids the loss of the liquid fibrin sealant by an active stream of bleeding.

Fibrin sealant can be used to assist with a wide variety of tissue apposition and adherence indications. The classic example is the use of fibrin sealant to eliminate potential spaces at the time of lymphatic dissections in the axilla or groin associated with tumor resections. The goal is to achieve adherence of the skin to underlying tissues after removal of lymphatics and soft tissue so that a potential space for seroma formation or bleeding is eliminated. Lymphatics and capillaries that are capable of contributing liquid to the space are also sealed. There are two major concepts that are important to understand when using fibrin sealant in this situation. First, there must be immediate contact between tissue layers during the period of fibrin sealant polymerization to achieve adherence. Second, once adherence is achieved, pulling the layers of tissue apart must be avoided to prevent mechanical disruption. Fibrin sealant is not an extremely strong adhesive, and this disruption can even be inadvertently performed. Unfortunately, if these two principles are not followed and a successful bonding of the layers is not achieved, one is left with a paradoxical antiadhesive effect. In essence, a layer of fibrin sealant that has completed its polymerization process and no longer will stick to tissues is left in place between the two layers. It acts like an antiadhesive, keeping the layers separate. This layer may potentiate the accumulation of fluids to a larger extent than if the sealant had not been used at all. The best technique to avoid the antiadhesive effects is to ensure immediate contact of the two surfaces. This can be done by first placing the latticework of sutures. For example, at the time of mastectomy and axillary dissection, if a preplaced latticework of skin sutures is created, it facilitates rapid wound closure. After placing latticework, fibrin sealant can be sprayed on the underlying muscle. Next, the latticework can be immediately tightened and the skin flaps can be closed with pressure applied on them to cause adherence between the skin and underlying muscle. After 2 to 3 minutes of pressure application during the polymerization of the fibrin sealant, the layers have become adherent. The capillaries and lymphatics are sealed. The potential space is eliminated. If, however, fibrin sealant is sprayed on the underlying muscle and a period of delay occurs while new sutures are placed to close the skin and then the skin is finally placed in contact with the underlying muscle after a period of multiple minutes, polymerization would be completed prior to contact of the skin and underlying muscle. In this setting, the fibrin sealant polymerization would be fully completed and the material would act as an antiadhesive, potentiating seroma formation. After achieving excellent adherence between the layers, it is important not to disrupt the bond by pulling up on the most superficial of the layers. Such disruption would again cause the fibrin sealant to function as an antiadhesive. The rapidity of fibrin sealant polymerization is dependent on the thrombin concentration. Thus, dilution of the thrombin component can produce a more slowly polymerizing material that will allow for less urgency in wound closure. It could also allow for careful and meticulous placement of a skin graft. This provides a time advantage that may be useful in some situations. However, in a situation in which significant variations in topography exist, liquid fibrin sealant tends to accumulate at the most dependent portions of the wound, particularly if it is polymerizing slowly. Thus, in this situation, it may be desirable to use the rapid wound closure techniques discussed and maintain the rapidly polymerizing concentration of thrombin so that fibrin sealant sticks quickly and covers the entire wound and does not accumulate at the most dependent portions of the operative field.

With respect to fistulae, whether they are bronchopleural, enterocutaneous, or other, a few principles are important to enhance the rate of successful closure with fibrin sealant. First the tract needs to be as clean as possible, and granulation tissue should be removed prior to placing the fibrin sealant. This is because moist, smooth surfaces are least likely to form adequate bonds with fibrin sealant. Removal of the granulation tissue is desirable, facilitating increased strength bonds with fibrin sealant and the highest likelihood of tract ablation. Second, the entire tract should be filled with fibrin sealant. It may be possible to facilitate this fibrin sealant placement by various imaging techniques. Computed tomography, fluoroscopy, and endoscopy can be employed to ensure that fibrin sealant is delivered throughout the fistula tract. Fibrin sealant closure of the tract is most likely to occur when the fistula tract is longer and has low output. It is less likely in a short tract that has high output. Thus, one can select those tracts that are most likely to be successfully closed by the guided application of fibrin sealant.

With respect to closure of pulmonary parenchymal air leaks, this is a challenging environment for fibrin sealant use. This is because the lung surface changes area on inspiration and expiration. Elasticity and strong adherence strength are required for the successful application of any adhesive to the surface of the lung. To achieve hemostasis, the fibrin sealant needs to be applied when there is no active air leak from the parenchymal surface. The lung needs to be deflated or softly clamped. After applying the fibrin sealant and 2 to 3 minutes of polymerization, reinflation can be permitted. It appears best to apply fibrin sealant to the lung in this setting using a spray technique. After polymerization is completed and reinflation occurs, the sealant will achieve hemostasis only if it is elastic enough to allow for the increased surface area of the lung with inflation and if the adherence strength is strong enough to maintain the adhesive surface bond to the lung. This setting is a significant mechanical challenge for the capacities of fibrin sealant.

Just as fibrin sealant is an excellent hemostatic agent for capillary and venous bleeding, it is also an excellent way to seal lymphatic vessels. The spray application of fibrin sealant to a lymphatic bed can achieve lymphostasis and prevent lymphocele formation. Some have suggested that aspiration of a lymphocele and replacement with fibrin sealant can also be used to treat established lymphoceles. At the time of a surgical operation, it is reasonable to apply the fibrin sealant to those areas in which active lymphatic leak is suspected or established. Clearly, the method will be successful only if the leaking lymphatics are treated. It is important to remember that the success of this treatment can be enhanced by achieving tissue apposition with layers of soft tissue over the lymphatic site using the rapid wound closure techniques described previously. This method not only will allow for lymphatic sealing but will also eliminate the potential space in which a lymphocele can accumulate.

SUMMARY

In this chapter, the history, mechanism of action, toxicity, clinical uses, and application techniques of fibrin sealant were reviewed. This widely useful material has been commercially available in the United States since 1998. The market for these products is expanding as surgeons gain increased experience with this agent. Future developments will include its use as a drug delivery and tissue engineering vehicle. New products are entering the marketplace, and safety and efficacy profiles are continuing to be improved by commercial manufacturers.

ACKNOWLEDGMENTS

We wish to thank Kristen Faircloth for her assistance in the preparation of this chapter.

REFERENCES

1. Spotnitz WD, Falstrom JK, Rodeheaver GT. The role of sutures and fibrin sealant in wound healing. Surg Clin North Am 1997;77:1–19.

2. Spotnitz WD. Introduction to special section on surgical tissue adhesives. Surgical tissue adhesives: new additions to the surgical armamentarium. J Long Term Effects Med Implants 2003;13:385–7.

3. Spotnitz WD. History of tissue adhesives. In: Sierra D, Saltz R, editors. Surgical adhesives and sealants: current technology and applications. Lancaster (PA): Technomic; 1996. p. 3–11.

4. Bergel S. Uber Wirkungen des Fibrins. Dtsch Med Wochenschr 1909;35:633.

5. Grey EG. Fibrin as a haomostatic in cerebral surgery. Surg Gynecol Obstet 1915;21:452–4.

6. Young JZ, Medawar PB. Fibrin suture of peripheral nerves. Lancet 1940;275:126–32.

7. Cronkite EP, Lozner EL, Deaver J. Use of thrombin and fibrinogen in skin grafting. JAMA 1944;124:976–8.

8. Matras H, Dings HP, Manoli B, et al. Zur nachtlosen Interfaszikularen Nerventransplantation im Tierexperiment. Wien Med Wochenschr 1972;122:517–23.

9. Gestring GF, Lerner R. Autologous fibrin for tissue-adhesion, hemostasis, and embolization. Vasc Surg 1983;17:294–304.

10. Siedentop KH, Harris DM, Sanchez B. Autologous fibrin tissue adhesive. Laryngoscope 1985;95:1074–6.

11. Spotnitz WD, Mintz PD, Avery N, et al. Fibrin glue from stored human plasma: an inexpensive and efficient method for local blood bank preparation. Am Surg 1987;53:460–4.

12. Schlag G, Redl H, editor. Fibrin sealing in surgical and nonsurgical fields. Vols 1–8. Berlin: Springer-Verlag; 1994.

13. Spotnitz WD. Fibrin sealant in the United States: clinical use at the University of Virginia. Thromb Haemost 1995;74:482–5.

14. Spotnitz, WD, Welker RL. Clinical uses of fibrin sealant. In: Mintz PD,

editor. Transfusion therapy: clinical principles and practice. Bethesda (MD): AABB Press; 1999. p. 199–222.

15. Rousou J, Gonzalez-Lavin L, Cosgrove D, et al. Randomized clinical trial of fibrin sealant in patients undergoing resternotomy or reoperation after cardiac operations. J Thorac Cardiovasc Surg 1989;97:194–203.

16. Sierra DH. Fibrin sealant adhesive systems: a review of their chemistry, material properties and clinical application. J Biomater Appl 1993;7:309–52.

17. Mosesson MW. Fibrinogen gamma chain functions. J Thromb Haemost 2003;1:231–8.

18. Pipan CM, Glasheen WP, Gonias SL, et al. Effects of antifibrinolytic agents on the life span of fibrin sealant. J Surg Res 1992;53:402–7.

19. Tisseel [package insert]. VH, Glendale (CA): Baxter Healthcare Corp.; November 2002.

20. Oswald A-M, Joly L-M, Gury C, et al. Fatal intraoperative anaphylaxis related to aprotinin after local application of fibrin glue. Anesthesiology 2003;99:521–3.

21. Busuttil RW. A comparison of antifibrinolytic agents used in hemostatic fibrin sealants. J Am Coll Surg 2003;197:1021–8.

22. Trasylol [package insert]. Glendale (CA): Bayer Pharmaeuticals Corp.; August 1998.

23. Crosseal [package insert]. Washington (DC): American Red Cross Blood Services; March 2003.

24. Schlag MG, Hopf R, Redl H. Convulsive seizures following subdural application of fibrin sealant containing tranexamic acid in a rat model. Neurosurgery 2000;47:1463–7.

25. Furtmuller R, Schlag MG, Berger M, et al. Tranexamic acid, a widely used antifibrinolytic agent causes convulsions by a X-aminoglutaric acid receptor antagonist effect. J Pharmacol Exp Ther 2002;301:168–73.

26. Schlag M, Hopf R, Redl H. Hind limb hyperexcitability following the application of a fibrin sealant containing tranexamic acid in the lumbar spinal cord in rats. Eur J Trauma 2002;28:252–7.

27. Schlag MG, Hopf R, Zifko U, Redl H. Epileptic seizures following cortical application of fibrin sealants containing tranexamic acid in rats. Acta Neurochir (Wien) 2002;144:63–9.

28. Spotnitz WD, Mintz PD, Avery N, et al. Fibrin glue from stored human plasma: an inexpensive and efficient method for local blood bank preparation. Am Surg 1987;53:460–4.

29. Siedentop K, Harris D, Ham K, et al. Extended experimental and preliminary surgical findings with autologous fibrin tissue adhesive made from patient's own blood. Laryngoscope 1986;96:1062–4.

30. Nichols WL, Daniels TM, Fisher PK. Antibodies to bovine thrombin and coagulation factor V associated with the use of topical bovine thrombin or fibrin glue: a frequent finding. Blood 1993;82:59a.

31. Ortel TL, Mercer MC, Thames EH, et al. Immunologic impact and clinical outcomes after surgical exposure to bovine thrombin. Ann Surg 2001;233:88–96.

32. Spotnitz WD, Burks, S. Use of tissue sealants in cardiac surgery. In: Franco KL, Verrier ED, editors. Advanced therapy in cardiac surgery. 2nd ed. Hamilton (ON): BC Decker Inc; 2003. p. 1–12.

33. Kjaergard HK, Fairbrother JE. Controlled clinical studies of fibrin sealant in cardiothoracic surgery—a review. Eur J Cardiothorac Surg 1996;10:727–33.

34. Hvass U, Chatel D, Frikha I, et al. Left ventricular free wall rupture: long-term results with pericardial patch and fibrin glue repair. Eur J Cardiothorac Surg 1995;9:75–6.

35. Kjaergard HK, Trumbull HR. Vivostat system autologous fibrin sealant: preliminary study in elective coronary bypass grafting. Ann Thorac Surg 1998;66:482–6.

36. Kjaergard HK, Trumbull HR. Bleeding from the sternal marrow can be stopped using Vivostat patient-derived fibrin sealant. Ann Thorac Surg 2000;69:1173–5.

37. Codispoti M, Mankad PS. Significant merits of a fibrin sealant in the presence of coagulopathy following paediatric cardiac surgery: randomized controlled trial. Eur J Cardiothorac Surg 2002;22:200–5.

38. Bayfield MS, Spotnitz WD. Fibrin sealant in thoracic surgery. Pulmonary applications, including management of bronchopleural fistula. Chest Surg Clin N Am 1996;6:576–83.

39. Wong K, Goldstraw P. Effect of fibrin glue in the reduction of post-thoracotomy alveolar air leak. Ann Thorac Surg 1997;64:979–81.

40. Fabian T, Federico JA, Ponn RB. Fibrin glue in pulmonary resection: a prospective, randomized, blinded study. Ann Thorac Surg 2003;75:1587–92.

41. Nomori H, Horio H, Suemasu K. Mixing collagen with fibrin glue to strengthen the sealing effect for pulmonary air leakage. Ann Thorac Surg 2000;70:1666–70.

42. Thistlethwaite PA, Luketich JD, Ferson PF, et al. Ablation of persistent air leaks after thoracic procedures with fibrin sealant. Ann Thorac Surg 1999;67:575–7.

43. Matthew TL, Spotnitz WD, Daniel TM, Kron IL. Closure of small bronchopleural fistulas using fibrin sealant through the flexible fiberoptic bronchoscope. Chest 1988;94:77S.

44. Takanami I. Closure of a bronchopleural fistula using a fibrin-glue coated collagen patch. Interact Cardiovasc Thorac Surg 2003;2:387–8.

45. Schenk W, Goldthwaite C Jr, Burks S, Spotnitz W. Fibrin sealant facilitates hemostasis in arteriovenous polytetrafluoroethylene grafts for

renal dialysis access. Am Surg 2002;68:728–32.

46. Schenk W, Burks S, Gagne P, et al. Fibrin sealant improves hemostasis in peripheral vascular surgery: a randomized prospective trial. Ann Surg 2003;237:871–6.

47. Kheirabadi BS, Pearson R, Rudnicka K, et al. Development of an animal model for assessment of the hemostatic efficacy of fibrin sealant in vascular surgery. J Surg Res 2001;100:84–92.

48. Padubidri AN, Browne E, Kononov A. Fibrin glue-assisted end-to-side anastomosis of rat femoral vessels: comparison with conventional suture method. Ann Plast Surg 1996;37:41–7.

49. Moskovitz MG, Bass L, Zhang L, Seibert JW. Microvascular anastomoses utilizing new intravascular stents. Ann Plast Surg 1994;32:612–8.

50. Drake DB, Faulkner BC, Amiss LR Jr, et al. Thrombogenic effects of a non thrombin-based fibrin sealant compared with thrombin-based fibrin sealant in microvenous anastomoses in a rat model. Ann Plast Surg 2000;45:520–4.

51. Frost-Armer L, Spotnitz WD, Rodeheaver GT, Drake DB. Comparison of the thrombogenicity of internationally available fibrin sealants in an established microsurgical model. J Plast Reconstruct Surg 2001;108:1655–60.

52. Zarge JI, Huang P, Husak V, et al. Fibrin glue containing fibroblast growth factor I and heparin with autologous endothelial cells reduces intimal hyperplasia in canine carotid artery balloon injury model. J Vasc Surg 1997;25:840–8.

53. Geissler HP, Gosselin C, Ren D, et al. Biointeractive polymers and tissue engineered blood vessels. Biomaterials 1996;17:329–36.

54. Stoker W, Nissen HW, Waldeau WR, et al. Perivenous application of fibrin glue reduces early injury of the human saphenous vein graft wall in an ex vivo model. Eur J Cardiothorac Surg 2002;21:212–7.

55. Lindsey WH, Masterson TM, Spotnitz WD, et al. Seroma prevention using fibrin glue in a rat model mastectomy rat model. Arch Surg 1990;125:305–7.

56. Moore MM, Nguyen DHD, Spotnitz WD. Fibrin sealant reduces serous drainage and allows earlier drain removal after axillary dissection: a randomized prospective trial. Am Surg 1997;63:97–102.

57. Kulber DA, Bacilious N, Peters ED, et al. The use of fibrin sealant in the prevention of seromas. Plast Reconstr Surg 1997;99:842–9.

58. Moore M, Burak W Jr, Nelson E, et al. Fibrin sealant reduces the duration and amount of fluid drainage following axillary dissection: a randomized prospective clinical trial. J Am Coll Surg 2001;192:591–9.

59. Langer S, Guenther JM, DiFronzo LA. Does fibrin sealant reduce drain output and allow earlier removal of drainage catheters in women undergoing operation for breast cancer? Am Surg 2003;69:77–81.

60. Medl M, Mayerhofer K, Peters-Engl E, et al. The application of fibrin glue after axillary lymphadenectomy in the surgical treatment of human breast cancer. Anticancer Res 1995;15:2843–6.

61. Dinsmore RC, Harris JA, Gustafson RJ. Effect of fibrin glue on lymphatic drainage after modifying radical mastectomy: a prospective randomized trial. Am Surg 2000;66:982–5.

62. MacPhee MJ, Campagna A, Best A, et al. Fibrin sealant as a delivery vehicle for sustained and controlled release of chemotherapy agents. In: Sierra D, Saltz R, editors. Surgical adhesives and sealants: current technology and applications. Lancaster (PA): Technomic; 1996. p. 145–54.

63. Miura S, Mii Y, Miyauchi Y, et al. Efficacy of slow-releasing anticancer drug delivery systems on transplantable osteosarcomas in rats. Jpn J Clin Oncol 1995;25:61–71.

64. Kitazawa H, Sata H, Adachi I, et al. Microdialysis assessment of fibrin glue containing sodium alginate for local delivery of doxorubicin in tumor-bearing rats. Biol Pharm Bull 1997;20:278–81.

65. Spotnitz WD, Burks S. The tissue adhesive decision; algorithm for successful clinical use.

66. Saltz R, Toriumi DM, editors. Tissue glues in cosmetic surgery. St. Louis (MO): Quality Medical, Inc; 2003. p. 46–67.

67. Spotnitz WD, Burks S. The tissue adhesive decision: algorithms for successful clinical use. In: Currie LJ, Sharpe JR, Martin R. The use of fibrin glue in skin grafts and tissue-engineered skin replacements: a review. Plast Reconstr Surg 2001;108:1718–26.

68. O'Grady KM, Agrawal A, Bhattacharyya TK, et al. An evaluation of fibrin tissue adhesive concentration and application thickness on skin graft survival. Laryngoscope 2000;110:1931–5.

69. Marchac D, Sandor G. Face lifts and sprayed fibrin glue: an outcome analysis of 200 patients. Br J Plast Surg 1994;47:306–9.

70. Shaffrey CI, Spotnitz WD, Shaffrey ME, Jane JA. Neurosurgical applications of fibrin glue: augmentation of dural closure in 134 patients. Neurosurgery 1990;26:207–10.

71. Patel MR, Louis W, Rachlin J. Postoperative cerebrospinal fluid leaks of the lumbosacral spine: management with percutaneous fibrin glue. AJNR Am J Neuroradiol 1996;17:495–500.

72. Ito S, Nagayama K, Iino N, et al. Frontal sinus repair with free autologous bone grafts and fibrin glue. Surg Neurol 2003;60:155–8.

73. Taguchi Y, Suzuki R, Okada M, Sekino H. Spinal arachnoid cyst developing after surgical treatment of a ruptured vertebral artery aneurysm: a possible complication of topical use of fibrin glue. J Neurosurg 1996;84:526–9.

74. Biedner B, Rosenthal G. Conjunctival closure in strabismus surgery: Vicryl versus fibrin glue. Ophthalmic Surg Lasers 1996;27:967.

75. Sharma A, Kaur R, Kumar S, et al. Fibrin glue versus n-butyl-2-cyanoacrylate in corneal perforations. Ophthalmology 2003;110:291–8.

76. Levy O, Martinowitz W, Oran A, et al. The use of fibrin tissue adhesive to reduce blood loss and the need for blood transfusion after total knee arthroplasty. J Bone Joint Surg Am 1999;81:1580–8.

77. Wang GJ, Hungerford DS, Savory CG, et al. Use of fibrin sealant to reduce bloody drainage and hemoglobin loss after total knee arthroplasty. A brief note of a randomized prospective trial. J Bone Joint Surg Am 2001;83-A:1503–5.

78. WangGJ, Goldthwaite CA Jr, Burks SG, Spotnitz WD. Experience improves successful use of fibrin sealant in total knee arthroplasty: implications for surgical education. J Long-Term Effects Med Implants 2003;13:389–97.

79. Wang GJ, Goldthwaite CA Jr, Burks SG, et al. Fibrin sealant reduces perioperative blood loss in total hip replacement. J Long-Term Effects Med Implants 2003;13:399–411.

80. Ochsner MG. Fibrin solutions to control hemorrhage in the trauma patient. J Long-Term Effects Med Implants 1998;8:161–73.

81. Larson MJ, Bowersox JC, Lim RC, Hess JR. Efficacy of a fibrin hemostatic bandage in controlling hemorrhage from experimental arterial injuries. Arch Surg 1995;130:420–2.

82. Holcomb JB, Pusateri AE, Hess JR, et al. Implications of new dry fibrin sealant technology for trauma surgery. Surg Clin North Am 1997;77:943–52.

83. Moralee SJ, Carney AS, Cash MP, Murray JAM. The effect of fibrin sealant haemostasis on post-operative pain in tonsillectomy. Clin Otolaryngol 1994;19:526–8.

84. Schlosser RJ, Gallagher R, Burks SG, et al. Autologous fibrin sealant reduces pain following tonsillectomy. Laryngoscope 2001;111:259–63.

85. Depondt J, Koka VN, Nasser T, et al. Use of fibrin glue in parotidectomy closure. Laryngoscope 1996;106:784–7.

86. Gleich LL, Rebeiz EE, Pankratov M, Shapshay SM. Autologous fibrin tissue adhesive in endoscopic sinus surgery. Otolaryngol Head Neck Surg 1995;112:238–41.

87. Vaiman M, Eviatar E, Segal S. Effectiveness of second-generation fibrin glue in endonasal operations. Otolaryngol Head Neck Surg 2002;126:388–91.

88. Bertrand B, Doyen A, Eloy P. Triosite implants and fibrin glue in the treatment of atrophic rhinitis: technique and results. Laryngoscope 1996;106:652–7.

89. Selesnick S, Mouwafak AR. Adhesives in otology and neurotology. Am J Otolaryngol 1997;18:81–9.

90. Daneshrad P, Chin GY, Rice DH. Fibrin glue presents complications of septal surgery: findings in a series of 100 patients. Ear Nose Throat J 2003;82:196–7.

91. Bar-Hava I, Krissi H, Ashkenazi J, et al. Fibrin glue improves pregnancy rates in women of advances reproductive age and in patients in whom in vitro fertilization attempts repeatedly fail. Fertil Steril 1999;71:821–4.

92. Kiilhoma P, Haarrala M, Polvi H, et al. Sutureless endoscopic colposuspension with fibrin sealant. Techn Urol 1996;1:81–3.

93. Phillippe HJ, Perdu M, Dompeyre P, et al. Transvaginal colpourethropexy with fibrin sealant: 4 years followup in 23 cases. Eur J Obstet Gynecol Reprod Biol 1996;70:157–8.

94. Young BK, Roque H, Abdelhak YE, et al. Minimally invasive endoscopy in the treatment of preterm premature rupture of membranes by application of fibrin sealant. J Perinat Med 2000;28:326–30.

95. Sciscione AC, Manley JS, Pollock M, et al. Intracervical fibrin sealants: a potential treatment for early preterm premature rupture of the membranes. Am J Obstet Gynecol 2001;184:368–73.

96. Reddy UM, Shah SS, Nemiroff RL, et al. In vitro sealing of punctured fetal membranes: potential treatment for midtrimester premature rupture of membranes. Am J Obstet Gynecol 2001;185:1090–3.

97. Janet L, Krizko M, Ferianec V, et al. Premature fetal membrane rupture after amniocentesis in the second trimester and successful use of fibrin glue—case report. Ceska Gynekol 2002;67:71–4.

98. Kumar U, Albala DM. Fibrin glue applications in urology. Curr Urol Rep 2001;2:79–82.

99. Shekarriz B, Stoller ML. The use of fibrin sealant in urology. J Urol 2002;167:1218–25.

100. Evans LA, Ferguson KH, Foley JP, et al. Fibrin sealant for the management of genitourinary injuries, fistulas and surgical complications. J Urol 2003;169:1360–2.

101. Valleix D, Descottes B. Pregluing of circular instrumental anastomoses. Surg Gynecol Obstet 1990;170:161–2.

102. Byrne DJ, Hardy J, Wood RAB, et al. Adverse influence of fibrin sealant on the healing of high-risk sutured colonic anastomoses. J R Coll Surg Edinb 1992;37:394–8.

103. van der Ham AC, Kort WJ, Weijma IM, et al. Effect of fibrin sealant on the integrity of colonic anastomoses in rats with faecal peritonitis. Eur J Surg 1993;159:427–32.

104. Detweiler MB, Verbo A, Kobos JW, et al. A sliding, absorbable, reinforced ring and an axially driven stent placement device for sutureless fibrin glue gastrointestinal anastomosis. J Invest Surg

1996;9:495–504.

105. Lau WY, Leung KL, Zhu XL, et al. Laparoscopic repair of perforated peptic ulcer. Br J Surg 1995;82:814–6.

106. Heneghan MA, Byrne A, Harrison PM. An open pilot study of the effects of a human fibrin glue for endoscopic treatment of patients with acute bleeding from gastric varices. Gastrointest Endosc 2002;56:422–6.

107. Datta D, Vlavianos P, Alisa A, Westaby D. Use of fibrin glue (Beriplast) in the management of bleeding gastric varices. Endoscopy 2003;35:675–8.

108. Imhof M, Ohmann C, Roher HD, Glutig H, DEUSUC Study Group. Endoscopic versus operative treatment in high-risk ulcer bleeding patients—results of a randomized study. Langenbecks Arch Surg 2003;387:327–36.

109. Pescatore P, Jornod P, Borovicka J, et al. Epinephrine versus epineph-rine plus fibrin glue injection in peptic ulcer bleeding: a prospective randomized trial. Gastrointest Endosc 2002;55:348–53.

110. Lin HJ, Hseih YH, Tseng GY, et al. Endoscopic injection with fibrin sealant versus epinephrine for arrest of peptic ulcer bleeding: a ran-domized, comparative trial. J Clin Gastroenterol 2002;35:218–21.

111. Cintron JR, Park JJ, Orsay CP, et al. Repair of fistulas-in-ano using fib-rin adhesive: long-term follow-up. Dis Colon Rectum 2000;43:944–9; discussion 949–50.

112. Lamont JP, Hooker G, Espenschied JR, et al. Closure of proximal col-orectal fistulas using fibrin sealant. Am Surg 2002;68:615–8.

113. Sentovich SM. Fibrin glue for anal fistulas: long-term results. Dis Colon Rectum 2003;46:498–502.

114. Zmora O, Mizrahi R, Rotholtz N, et al. Fibrin glue sealing in the treat-ment of perineal fistulas. Dis Colon Rectum 2003;46:584–9.

115. Buchanan GN, Bertram CI, Phillips RK, et al. Efficacy of fibrin sealant in the management of complex anal fistula: a prospective trial. Dis Colon Rectum 2003;49:1167–74.

116. Aitola P, Hiltunen KM, Matikainen M. Fibrin glue in perianal fistu-las—a pilot study. Ann Chir Gynaecol 1999;88:136–8.

117. Rakocz M, Mazar A, Varon D, et al. Dental extractions in patients with bleeding disorders. Oral Surg Oral Med Oral Pathol 1993;75:280–2.

118. Rakocz M, Lavie G, Martinowitz W. Glanzmann's thrombasthenia: the use of autologous fibrin glue in tooth extractions. ASDC J Dent Child 1995;62:129–31.

119. Yucel EA, Oral O, Olgac V, Oral CK. Effects of fibrin glue on wound healing in oral cavity. J Dent 2003;31:569–75.

120. Trombelli L, Schincaglia GP, Zangari F, et al. Effects of tetracycline HCI conditioning and fibrin-fibronectin system application in the treat-ment of buccal gingival recession with guided tissue regeneration. J

Periodontol 1995;66:313–20.

121. Trombelli L, Scabbia A, Wikesjo UM, Calura G. Fibrin glue application in conjunction with tetracycline root conditioning and coronally positioned flap procedure in the treatment of human gingival recession defects. J Clin Periodontol 1996;23:861–77.

122. Trombelli L, Scabbia A, Scapoli C, Calura G. Clinical effect of tetracycline demineralization and fibrin-fibronectin sealing system application on healing response following flap débridement surgery. J Periodontol 1996;67:688–93.

123. Singh MP, Brady R Jr, Drohan W, MacPhee MJ. Sustained release of antibiotics from fibrin sealant. In: Sierra D, Saltz R, editors. Surgical adhesives and sealants: current technology and applications. Lancaster (PA): Technomic; 1996. p. 121–33.

124. MacPhee MH, Singh MP, Brady R Jr, et al. Fibrin sealant: a versatile delivery vehicle for drugs and biologics. In: Sierra D, Saltz R, editors. Surgical adhesives and sealants: current technology and applications. Lancaster (PA): Technomic; 1996. p. 109–20.

125. Kitajiri S, Tabuchi K, Hiraumi H, Kaetsu H. Relief of post-tonsillectomy pain by release of lidocaine from fibrin glue. Laryngoscope 2001;111:642–4.

126. Marone P, Monzillo V, Segu C, Antoniazzi E. Antibiotic-impregnated fibrin glue in ocular surgery: in vitro antibacterial activity. Ophthalmologica 1999;213:12–5.

127. Woolverton CJ, Fulton JA, Salstrom SJ, et al. Tetracycline delivery from fibrin controls peritoneal infection without measurable systemic antibiotic. J Antimicrob Chemother 2001;48:861–7.

128. Mader JT, Stevens CM, Stevens JH, et al. Treatment of experimental osteomyelitis with a fibrin sealant antibiotic implant. Clin Orthop 2002;403:58–72.

129. Iwaya K, Mizoi K, Tessler A, Itoh Y. Neurotrophic agents in fibrin glue mediate adult dorsal root regeneration into spinal cord. Neurosurgery 1999;44:589–95.

130. Yin Q, Kemp GJ, Yu LG, et al. Neurotrophin-4 delivered by fibrin glue promotes peripheral nerve regeneration. Muscle Nerve 2001;24:345–51.

131. Bannasch H, Horch RE, Tanczos E, Stark GB. Treatment of chronic wounds with cultured autologous keratinocytes as suspension in fibrin glue. Zentralbl Chir 2000;125 Suppl 1:79–81.

132. Cohen M, Bahoric A, Clarke HM. Aerosolization of epidermal cells with fibrin glue for the epithelialization of porcine wounds with unfavorable topography. Plast Reconstr Surg 2001;107:1208–15.

133. Currie LJ, Sharpe JR, Martin R. The use of fibrin glue in skin grafts and tissue-engineered skin replacements: a review. Plast Reconstr Surg 2001;108:1713–26.

134. van Susante JL, Buma P, Schuman L, et al. Resurfacing potential of het-

erologous chondrocytes suspended in fibrin glue in large full-thickness defects of femoral articular cartilage: an experimental study in the goat. Biomaterials 1999;20:1167–75.

135. Tholpady SS, Schlosser R, Spotnitz W, et al. Repair of an osseous facial critical-size defect using augmented fibrin sealant. Laryngoscope 1999;109:1585–8.

136. Cederholm-Williams SA. Therapeutic use of fibrin—a new class of fibrin sealant with minimal risks. Ukr Biokhim Zh 1996;68:34–6.

137. CryoSeal [panel brochure]. Sacramento (CA): AHE Thermogenesis Corp.; 1999.

5 Protein Polymers

K. ÜMIT YÜKSEL, PhD

Advances in surgery have necessitated the development of new approaches to surgical procedures. The use of surgical adhesives to glue incised or torn tissue and to seal anastomotic leaks, whether these are the anastomoses of the airways, vasculature, or organs such as the pancreas, has contributed to this advancement. This chapter reviews the biology, chemistry, resorption, and clinical uses of two products, CoSeal Surgical Sealant (Cohesion Technologies, Inc./Baxter Healthcare International, Palo Alto, CA) and BioGlue Surgical Adhesive (CryoLife, Inc., Kennesaw, GA). Both have been approved for clinical use in the United States, European Union, and elsewhere and are in extensive clinical use. Although their initial and primary use was sealing of vascular anastomoses, their utility and regulatory approvals have gone far beyond that.

HISTORY AND BACKGROUND

The use of proteins as bonding agents is quite an ancient matter. Egg white, which is predominantly ovalbumin, was used as a binding agent in construction and sculptures during the Middle Ages. Glues made from animal hides are still used in woodworking. The use of proteins as surgical adhesives dawned in the twentieth century with the fibrin-based adhesives, described elsewhere in this book. An in-depth review of the history of fibrin-thrombin– or thrombin-based tissue sealants and their clinical use in plastic surgery was recently published as a book.[1]

The subjects of this chapter are adhesives and sealants that use cross-linking agents and covalently bind to tissue surfaces. The most significant difference of this class of adhesives and sealants from the fibrin-thrombin–based sealants is their independence of the coagulation cascade. These sealants function independently of the coagulation state (coagulopathic or anticoagulated) of the patient. A comprehensive but nonexhaustive list of this dynamic field can be found in Table 5–1.

A surgical adhesive with a cross-linking agent was initially developed at the Batelle Memorial Institute. Its experimental use was described by Braunwald and colleagues.[2,3] This product, known as GRF-glue (gelatin, resorcinol, formaldehyde) (manufactured by Cardial SA, Saint Etienne, France, as well as other companies), remained dormant until it was rediscovered by a group of French surgeons, who pioneered its clinical use by extensively and successfully applying it for the treatment of aortic dissections. They published their progress in a series of manuscripts,[4,5] including a 20-year follow-up on their work.[6] This frequent clinical use by the French surgeons earned it the nickname "French glue." The GRF-glue consists of two solutions, one containing the resorcinol and gelatin mixture and the other the formaldehyde solution. Prior to application, the gelatin-resorcinol component is warmed to 40°C to melt it. It is used primarily in Europe for repair of aortic dissections and is not available in the United States.

A similar adhesive (GR-Dial, Fehling, Germany) containing gelatin, resorcinol, and a mixture of oxaldehyde and glutaraldehyde, instead of formaldehyde, which is primarily available in Germany, was reported by Ennker and colleagues and Wertzel and colleagues.[7,8] This adhesive was reported to bind through the polycondensation reaction of aldehyde groups with the alcohol groups from resorcinol (1,3–benzenediol). Others have also published on the experimental use of yet another variation of the GRF-glue for sealing air leaks from lungs.[9,10]

FocalSeal-L Synthetic Absorbable Sealant (Focal Inc., Massachusetts, USA) became the first surgical adhesive with a cross-linking agent to be approved by the US Food and Drug Administration (FDA) for clinical use. FocalSeal-L also bears the CE-Mark, and in the European literature, it is known as AdvaSeal. It is based on polyethylene glycol (PEG) macromonomers derivatized with functional groups

Table 5–1 Chemical Composition of Surgical Adhesives of Sealants Using Cross-linking Agents

Brand Name	Manufacturer	Composition	CE-Mark	FDA Status	FDA Indication
GRF	Cardial SA (France)	Gelatin, resorcinol, formaldehyde	Yes	None	None
GR-Dial	Fehling (Germany)	Gelatin, resorcinol, oxaldehyde, glutaraldehyde	?	None	None
FocalSeal	Genzyme BioSurgery (USA)	Functionalized PEG polymer and eosin-Y	Yes	Approved	Sealing of air leaks from lungs*
BioGlue	CryoLife Inc. (USA)	Albumin and glutaraldehyde	Yes	Approved	Tissue bonding and vascular sealing*
CoSeal	Cohesion Technologies Inc. (USA)	Two functionalized, 4-armed PEGs	Yes	Approved	Sealing suture lines*
DuraSeal	Confluent Surgical Inc (USA)	Two functionalized, multiarmed PEGs	Yes	IDE[†]	Sealing of CSF leaks[‡]
TissueBond	TissueMed (UK)	Albumin, methylene blue	Yes	None	None
Not commercially available	3M (USA)	Albumin and functionalized PEG [43]	?	PMA[§]	Sealing of air leaks from lungs[44][‡]
Thorex	Surgical Sealants Inc. (USA)	Albumin, carbodiimide, surfactant, and lipid[45]	No	IDE	Sealing of air leaks from lungs[‡]
Not commercially available	PPTI (USA)	Recombinant peptides and glutaraldehyde	No	IDE	Urinary stress incontinence[‡]

FDA = US Food and Drug Administration; IDE = investigational drug exemption; PMA = premarketing approval.
*Specific wording of the indications can be found on the FDA Web site (<http://www.fda.gov>) and on the instructions for use provided with each product.
[†]Granted for clinical trial.
[‡]Exact wording of the indications is determined at the premarketing approval stage, following the clinical trial.
[§]Filed with the FDA.

(diacrylate esters). These polymers are cross-linked with each other via light activation.[11,12] The product is currently manufactured and distributed by Genzyme BioSurgery (Lexington, MA) and is the only sealant approved specifically and solely for sealing of air leaks during lung surgery. The product kit consists of several liquid components that are applied (brushed on and allowed to penetrate the tissue) in sequence and then polymerized by shining light onto the site from an external light source. The kit is stored frozen (–20°C) and is thawed before use. The published literature indicates that this product acts as a mechanical leakage barrier for 14 days and was still detectable without any cellular ingrowth at 6 weeks.[11]

BioGlue Surgical Adhesive and CoSeal Surgical Sealant were the next products of this class to be approved by the FDA. They also bear the CE-Mark for various indications, which are discussed in detail in this chapter. Both products are for single-patient use only and may not be resterilized.

CoSeal Surgical Sealant is provided as a sterile kit stored at room temperature (25°C). Currently, the kit contains one syringe filled with a functionalized PEG polymer solution, one syringe with another functionalized PEG polymer powder, and a syringe containing the solvent. After the powder is dissolved, the syringes containing the two PEG polymer solutions are assembled into a delivery device. The manufacturer recommends that the unit be used within 2 hours of preparation. The material is applied through either an applicator tip or a spray device (Figure 5–1).

BioGlue Surgical Adhesive is provided in a sterile kit with the albumin (45% w/v) and glutaraldehyde (10% w/v) solutions prefilled into a two-barrel cartridge, which is stored at room temperature (< 25°C). The room temperature–stored ready-to-use solutions eliminate any need or time for preparation. The cartridge is inserted into a resterilizable delivery device, and the material is applied to the surgical site through a mixing tip that attaches to the cartridge. Applicator tips of multiple lengths are provided to facilitate its use during surgery. Given that the components are in their final state at the time of manufacture, there is no recommended time limitation on the use of the assembled kit (Figure 5–2).

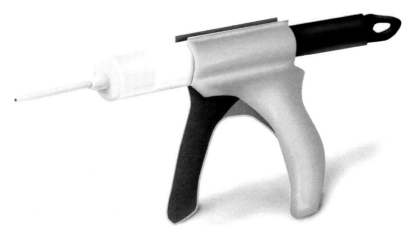

■ FIGURE 5–1   Fully prepared CoSeal applicator ready for use.

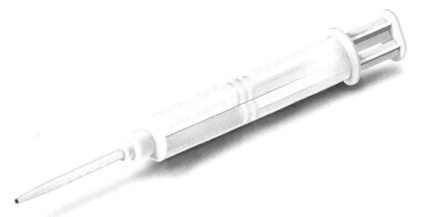

■ FIGURE 5–2   Fully prepared BioGlue applicator ready for use.

REGULATION

Both BioGlue and CoSeal are classified and regulated as medical devices in the United States and European Union. As such, they have obtained Pre-Market Approval (PMA) from the FDA and a CE-Mark from a notified body in the European Union (for the regulatory status of others, see Table 5-1). The PMA is granted after an extensive evaluation of a clinical study conducted on humans receiving the treatment under investigation. Medical devices are also subject to postmarket surveillance, which consists of reporting and collecting adverse events, both under the FDA and European Union systems. The FDA adverse event report database for all medical devices, including these two sealants, is available on the World Wide Web at <http://www.fda.gov/cdrh/maude>.

CHEMISTRY AND POLYMERIZATION

As described above, both CoSeal and BioGlue are members of a family of surgical sealants and adhesives that use cross-linking agents. The common theme for this type of adhesives is the presence of a matrix and a cross-linking agent. The matrix is a protein, a peptide, or an inert synthetic polymer that has been subsequently functionalized. The common functional group on the proteins is an amine group. Other functional groups for the matrix or the cross-linking agent include aldehyde, anhydride, succinimide, or thiol groups that are part of a small (eg, glutaraldehyde) or a large (eg, PEG macromer) molecule. The composition of this family is detailed in Table 5-1.

The generalized chemical reactions for BioGlue and CoSeal are shown in Figure 5–3. Both of these reactions are chemically similar to each other (nucleophilic attack of the amine or thiol to the succinimide or aldehyde), even if the macromers are structurally different from each other.

The cross-linking of BioGlue to itself and to the tissue is the result of the reaction between the amine groups and aldehyde groups. The aldehyde groups are provided by the bifunctional reagent glutaraldehyde. The amine groups come from the side chains of the lysine residues of the albumin. There are 59 lysines in bovine serum albumin, which provides a maximum of one cross-link per ~ 10 amino acids, or ~ 1,100 Da molecular weight. Although this material is designed to covalently bind to proteins, it will also nonspecifically bind to other substances. Substances containing amine groups will experience the same chemical binding as proteins. Items that are not proteinaceous in nature (such as gauze or forceps) may be adhered to by physical forces as the material polymerizes in their microscopic surface crevices. A similar observation has also been reported for CoSeal.[13]

CoSeal consists of two different tetrafunctional PEG macromers, which are, by simplest description, cross-shaped.[14] PEG polymers of ~ 2,500 Da molecular weight are bound to a central molecule (pentaerytritol), resulting in a macromer of ~ 10,000 Da. These macromers are then derivatized with reactive groups such as succinimidylglutarate and thiol at their termini.[15] When dissolved in buffers of appropriate pH and mixed with each other, these macromers react with each other and form a gel. The end product was proposed to be a thioester, and N–hydroxysuccinimide, another reactive compound,

A

B

■ FIGURE 5–3   (*A*) Reaction mechanisms of BioGlue and CoSeal. Reaction of a tetrafunctional succinimdylglutaryl polyethylene glycol (PEG) macromer with a thiol PEG macromer (left) and a protein (right) to form a dimer, which leads to cross-linked polymers. (*B*) Progressive reaction of glutaraldehyde with bovine serum albumin (BSA) (shown as R4) and cell surface proteins (shown as R5) to form dimers and polymers.

was proposed as the side product.[14] The thio- and carboxyester bonds were proposed to be the labile bonds leading to the hydrolysis of the gel. It was also noted that the macromer solutions themselves are subject to simple hydrolysis or oxidation before they are mixed with each other.

DEGRADATION

Both BioGlue and CoSeal are degraded in the body after implantation. Their degradation rates and mechanisms are different from each other.

The thioester and carboxyester bonds in CoSeal were identified as the labile sites.[14] The gel was reported to dissolve in vitro after several days after incubation at 37°C in buffer via the hydrolysis of these bonds on reaction with water. This hydrolytic degradation may, in part, be responsible for the swelling of the polymer once it is implanted. An in vitro swell ratio of 4.3 ± 0.6 (4.3 times swelling of its original volume) was also reported.[14] In vivo, CoSeal reportedly degraded within < 30 days of implantation and could not be discerned grossly or histologically at 30 days.[13]

The major component of BioGlue is albumin, an abundant natural protein. Therefore, it is degraded by proteolysis, the enzymatic breakdown and removal of proteins. The proteases are furnished by lysosomes and macrophages, which specialize in protein degradation. Because albumin is a natural protein, BioGlue is resorbed slowly. Histologically, the material was detectable after 1 year in a goat model.[16] The initial observation of resorption was in a long-term (24 months) vascular implant in sheep. The 24-month sheep explant showed a range of phases of the remodeling of the BioGlue implant. Most regions exhibited minimal inflammatory activity (regions of encapsulation), whereas others showed signs of resorption. Cells infiltrated BioGlue as the resorption process evolved, laying down collagen as part of the normal healing process.[17] Since that original report, human explants with different dwell times have been examined and were found to show a similar remodeling reaction (CW Hewitt, personal communication, 2003).

TOXICITY AND BIOCOMPATIBILITY

By definition, all of the medical devices approved for clinical use in the United States or European Union are evaluated for biocompatibility for their intended use. Regulatory bodies in the United States, European Union, Canada, Japan, and elsewhere require that all medical devices are biocompatible. The manufacturers must submit their candidate devices to a series of biocompatibility tests, summarized under the International Standards Organization (ISO) 10993 guidance document. This panel of tests includes general toxicity, cytotoxicity, and mutagenicity studies. All of these tests must be completed before a medical device is approved. In addition, before any medical device is implanted in humans, a series of tests are conducted in animals to show the clinical utility of the candidate device.

The biocompatibility of medical devices also involves their delivery systems. All product-contacting components are United States Pharmacopeia (USP) class VI compliant, which, by definition, have been tested and demonstrated to be biocompatible and nontoxic.

Although these products have been determined to be safe for the indications and dosage for which they are approved, surgeons must pay close attention to the Instructions for Use (IFU) included with each product. They need to be very studious and careful if their applications take them outside the approved indications. Such deviations may include and have included excessive volume applied or delivery into closed spaces, both of which have resulted in pressure on and temporary impairment of nerves.

BioGlue and CoSeal contain reactive molecules to perform their intended function. These molecules will react with the other components of the product and with the tissue proteins. Both products adhere to tissue proteins by covalent chemical bonds. This means that there is a chemical reaction between the product and tissue surface. Once implanted, there will be some foreign-body reaction to the implanted material.[13,17] The extent of the foreign-body reaction may be different for each product and may depend on the site of implantation and on the individual person in whom the material is implanted. Although not proven, it may also be technique dependent. The difference in the observed reaction is exemplified by three separate publications, two of which found a minimal inflammatory response,[14,16] whereas the third reported a greater response.[18]

EFFECTIVENESS

The ability of CoSeal to inhibit suture line bleeding was evaluated in a canine iliac polytetrafluoroethylene (PTFE) graft model.[13] It was reported to significantly reduce the time to hemostasis (on average 302 ± 357 s vs > 900 s; $p < .05$) and volume of blood lost (19 ± 34 g vs 284 ± 151 g; $p < .05$) when compared with tamponade as the control group.

The clinical effectiveness of CoSeal for sealing peripheral arterial and/or venous reconstructions was evaluated in two clinical studies.

The US study was a prospective, randomized, controlled multicenter ($N = 9$ participating sites) trial with 148 patients, half of which were treated with CoSeal and the other half with the control substance (absorbable gelatin sponge and thrombin hemostat; Gelfoam [Pharmacia-Upjohn, Kalamazoo, MI] and thrombin).[19] This study was designed to evaluate whether the success rate for the experimental treatment was equivalent to that of the control. The overall number of treated sites was 136 for the experimental group and 128 for the control group. The most common surgical procedures involved were infrainguinal revascularization (35–39%) and dialysis access shunts (58–59%). The primary measure of success was the cessation of bleeding at a treatment site within 600 seconds. The secondary measure was the time to sealing, that is, the duration from restoration of circulation to the graft to cessation of bleeding. This study demonstrated that the CoSeal was equivalent to the control treatment whether or not the data were analyzed on a per-patient basis (86% vs 80%; $p = .29$). The benefit of the experimental treatment was more obvious from the secondary measure of success (16.5 seconds vs 189 seconds; $p = .01$). This was partially due to a larger fraction of patients achieving immediate sealing (0 seconds) in the CoSeal group (47% vs 20%; $p < .001$). This was the pivotal study for the evaluation of the product in the United States (Figure 5–4).

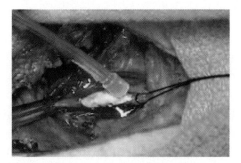

■ FIGURE 5–4   CoSeal used to seal the suture lines and reinforce a vascular patch of the carotid artery.

A multicenter, nonrandomized clinical study evaluated the performance of CoSeal in sealing suture lines along synthetic (Dacron and PTFE) and autologous vein grafts on 131 patients in Europe. The overall success rate for achieving sealing was 85%. The rates of success for PTFE, Dacron, and autologous vein graft materials were 74%, 95%, and 96%, respectively.[20]

The clinical utility of BioGlue was initially evaluated in an ovine model for surgical repair of aortic dissections. A descending aortic dissection was created in sheep. The animals were then randomized in a blinded fashion to surgical repair or surgical repair plus gluing the layers of the dissection with BioGlue.[21] The results revealed that BioGlue decreased the incidence of (1) acute postrepair rupture of the aorta from 30 to 0%, (2) redissection at the site of distal surgical repair from 17 to 0%, (3) dissection progression prior to healing from 17 to 0%, and (4) chronic dissection formation from 75 to 0% in animals surviving 90 days (planned end point) (Figure 5–5).

The utility of BioGlue as an anastomotic sealant of large-diameter synthetic grafts was evaluated in coagulopathic sheep against Surgicel (Johnson & Johnson, Somerville, NJ). Postsurgical bleeding was significantly less in the BioGlue group compared with controls (995 vs 470 mL; $p < .003$).[17]

The clinical effectiveness of BioGlue was initially evaluated in 175 patients (54 nonrandomized [lead-in] patients, 60 patients randomized to standard surgery plus BioGlue, and 61 patients randomized to standard surgery only). An interim analysis was performed on the randomized portion of the trial, which showed no statistically significant difference in early mortality (primary end point) between the two groups; however, BioGlue–treated patients required fewer pledgets, hemostatic agents, and makeup stitches than the patients in the control group. This led the FDA to grant a Humanitarian Device Exemption (HDE) in December 1999 as the initial US approval for

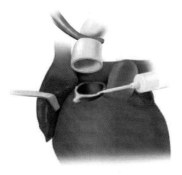

■ FIGURE 5–5 BioGlue used to reinforce the repair of an aortic dissection.

the use of BioGlue as an adjunct in the surgical repair of acute thoracic aortic dissections.

Subsequently, the clinical effectiveness of BioGlue as a surgical adjunct in cardiac and vascular surgical repairs was evaluated in a prospective, multicenter, randomized, controlled trial involving 151 patients.[22] Patients were randomized to receive standard surgical repair with BioGlue applied to the anastomotic site prior to clamp removal (BioGlue group, $n = 76$), or standard surgical anastomotic repair alone (control group, $n = 75$). The hypothesis was that hemostasis would be achieved in a higher percentage (superiority, not equivalence) of the BioGlue–treated patients than in the control patients. Surgical procedures encountered in this trial included cardiac, aortic, and peripheral vascular procedures (22.6, 53.8, and 23.6% for the BioGlue group and 26.3, 49.5, and 24.2% for the control group). The primary end point was the achievement of anastomotic hemostasis, which was a simple "yes" or "no" answer. Anastomotic hemostasis was defined as an anastomosis that did not require additional agents (pledgets, sutures, hemostatic devices, antifibrinolytic agents, thrombin glues, fibrin glues) at the treated site(s) to control bleeding at any point during the course of the original operation. Secondary evaluations included the number of donor exposures of blood replacement products administered and the type of additional agents used (pledgets, sutures, hemostatic devices, antifibrinolytic agents, thrombin glues, fibrin glues). The effectiveness of BioGlue was shown on both a per-patient (61% vs 39%; $p = .014$) and a per-anastomosis basis (81% vs 57%; $p < .003$). There were no significant differences in the secondary evaluation points, except that the number of neurologic deficits was less for the BioGlue group (6.5%) than for the control group (21.6%; $p = .009$) and the incidence of adjunctive pledget use on their primary repairs to achieve hemostasis ($p < .05$) was lower.[22] This led to a PMA in December 2001 for use in vascular repair.

Because both of these products were approved only in December 2001, the number of publications on the different clinical applications of CoSeal and BioGlue is limited. The FDA's *Manufacturer and User Facility Device Experience Database* (MAUDE) serves as a source for surgeons to learn what other clinical applications these products are being used for and what the pitfalls are. For example, from this database, one learns that both products have been used for sealing the dural leaks in spinal or cranial surgery. In the case of CoSeal, we also learn that this product may swell four to five times its dispensed volume, which may cause unintended side effects if placed in a confined environment. In the case of BioGlue, we learn about clinical uses outside the United States and that cerebrospinal fluid leaks may recur (in one case after 3 days, in another 2 months after surgery). These examples should serve as a caution to surgeons about the proper uses of these devices.

CLINICAL USES

The clinical indications approved for these products, along with contraindications, precautions, and warnings, are listed in the current versions of their IFU. Please note that IFUs are living documents that are revised periodically based on either the feedback received from the health care professionals who use these devices, additional studies carried out by their manufacturers, adverse events reported, or information gained otherwise. The approved indications for use in the United States, European Union, and the rest of the world are not always consistent with each other, with the US indications usually lagging behind owing to more stringent requirements for regulatory approval. For example, BioGlue is approved for use as an adjunct to standard methods of achieving hemostasis in adult patients in open surgical repair of large vessels in the United States, but it is approved more broadly for soft tissue repair (including sealing air leaks from surgical lung repairs) under the CE-Mark in the European Union and elsewhere. The literature documents uses of these products in various areas. One is reminded, however, that both of these devices are intended for use on the outside of the blood vessels, not on the inside. These devices are to be used as adjuncts to conventional methods of closure, such as sutures and staples, not as their replacements.

CoSeal is indicated for use in vascular reconstructions to achieve adjunctive hemostasis by mechanically sealing areas of leakage. No contraindications were listed for this device in the initial approval. Subsequently, a warning was added to the labeling regarding swell volumes of the sealant.[23] This swell volume is reported to be four- to fivefold in vivo, and surgeons are advised that CoSeal does swell and should not be placed in any anatomic area in which swelling can lead to a compression problem. The in vivo swell volume is consistent with that reported (see above) in vitro. Swelling of BioGlue has not been reported.

In a rabbit epicardial abrasion model, CoSeal was compared with surgical control and Tissucol (Baxter Healthcare S.A.S.; Maurepas, France) for preventing adhesions of the pericardium to the surrounding tissue.[24] CoSeal reduced the tenacity and extent of adhesions over both comparison groups. Subsequently, it has been marketed in Europe under the trade name Adhibit for the prevention of adhesions at surgical sites. It has been CE-Marked for this purpose. In a very limited series of patients, the material was shown to reduce the extent and severity of adhesions threefold ($p < .01$) in infants undergoing staged surgical correction of congenital heart abnormalities.[25]

Reported uses of BioGlue are summarized below.[26-35] The article by Coselli and colleagues is especially illustrative of the surgical technique for aortic dissection repair.[27] Fink and colleagues published detailed drawings showing different surgical techniques for cardiac repair.[30] BioGlue has also been used for sealing air and fluid leaks. Herget and colleagues originally demonstrated its utility for sealing air leaks in sheep.[31] Sealing of air leaks from parenchyma or bronchial anastomoses was immediate. Lai and colleagues reported the initial clinical uses for sealing air leaks.[32] Recently, BioGlue was reported to reduce the air leak duration (0.42 vs 3.68 days; $p < .001$) and median chest tube drainage time (2.33 vs 5.42 days; $p < .05$) in a series of 21 patients undergoing treatment for bullectomy.[33] More recently, its successful use in sealing bronchopleural fistulae has been described.[34] It has also been used for prevention of cerebrospinal fluid leaks in neurosurgical procedures ($N = 216$ procedures) in which watertight closure of the dura mater could not be achieved by primary suture alone and for reconstruction of the sellar floor following transsphenoidal adenohypophysectomy. These included supratentorial (52.7%) and infratentorial (24.5%) craniotomies, transsphenoidal adenohypophysectomies (18.9%), and spinal (3.7%) procedures.[35] Such procedures require the utmost attention of the surgeon because one animal study demonstrated nerve damage when BioGlue was applied onto exposed nerves.[36] The same authors found that nerves can be protected by the use of surgical lubricants.[37]

COST

The costs of these products vary with the markets in which they are sold. In the United States, their cost is estimated to range from $50 to $135/mL, depending on the size of the unit (2, 5, or 10 mL fill volumes for BioGlue; 2, 4, or 8 mL fill volumes for CoSeal). These values are comparable to fibrin sealants ($50 to $120 per mL; 1, 2, or 5 mL fill volume). Surgical adhesives and sealants are reimbursed by insurance companies and the like. Although these products may add to the list cost of the surgery, they may also reduce the cost of surgery if leak-free anastomoses lead to a shorter operating time (average operating time cost of $500/15 min) and early discharge from the hospital. Proving such a cost savings may be difficult because most of these patients have other associated comorbidities. The cost benefit may also not be realized in regions where blood products ($50 for platelets to $115 for fresh frozen plasma; 2002 Medicare reimbursement prices in the United States) are not charged to the patient or the hospital. However, another cost savings may arise from the reduced exposure of the patient to transfused blood products. The cost-effectiveness of surgical sealants has been discussed by others as well.[22]

APPLICATION TECHNIQUES

Both BioGlue and CoSeal are applied as liquids that polymerize rapidly to a hydrogel. By definition, hydrogels have a high water content and readily absorb or release water. The human body is a form of hydrogel, with an average water content of 70%. Therefore, these two products will remain flexible and pliable while hydrated inside the human body. They will, however, desiccate and may harden if left exposed to the environment (air) for a long period.

All surgical adhesives and sealants have at least a few days of dwell time. This is also true for fibrin sealants. In this respect, surgical adhesives and sealants are like a suture, vascular graft, or any other material that is implanted. They will occupy a space. If the surrounding tissue is closed tightly over these items after their application, the added material will apply pressure to the surrounding tissue. If the application is made onto a blood vessel, the implant may compress on it and alter the flow dynamics. The thicker the applied layer is, the greater the impediment may be. Other hemostatic agents are also known to cause similar artifacts.

In many respects, surgical adhesives are not very different from their industrial or household adhesives. For example, all of these require a clean field for a strong bond. For household and industrial adhesives, the interfering substance may be grease or sawdust; for surgical adhesives, it is blood or blood clot. CoSeal and BioGlue rely on the reactions of amines and thiols, which are amply present in proteins. Blood is a very rich source of protein. If the field is not free from blood or blood clot, these adhesives will bind to blood proteins instead of the underlying tissue. This will lead to an unsatisfactory outcome, that is, continued bleeding or recurrence of bleeding.

Obtaining a clean or dry field before applying these products should improve the desired outcome.

Another commonality of adhesives is that they work better when applied as a thin film, not as a thick layer. Unlike adding yet another suture to stop bleeding, adding another thick layer of an adhesive may not be better. Thickness is a relative concept. In this case, the scale is in millimeters, not centimeters. In contrast to pharmaceutical agents, there is no prescribed dosage for the use of surgical adhesives. Nevertheless, there are recommendations by the manufacturers to apply thin layers, and the IFU mention the maximum amount of material implanted during clinical trials. It is simple to calculate how much material one might expect to use at the site of application. For example, if one is sealing a vessel with a 6 mm outer diameter and the sealant is applied circumferentially 10 mm on either side of the suture line to a thickness of 2 mm, one expects to use 1 mL of product. Similarly, a suture line of 5 cm length coated 1 cm wide on either side to a thickness of 1 mm would require 1 mL material. If a larger amount of material is used, one should suspect that the material is flowing away from where it is applied, is coating the surrounding tissue, or is pooling below the site of application. The values used here, especially the thickness of the material applied, are for illustration purposes only. This is neither medical advice nor a recommendation on how to use any of these products. It is simple mathematics that can guide one's expectations of how much material to use.

As any chemical reaction, the cross-linking (ie, gelation) of these products is temperature dependent and will be retarded by the lower temperature of the product. Because neither is an exothermic reaction, in contrast to bone cement (methacrylate), the polymerization reaction will not be accelerated by the heat generated. The lack of heat generated enhances the biocompatibility of both products because the adjacent tissue is not affected. On the other hand, if the product is cold, it may take longer for the gelation reaction to be complete.

Application techniques are not limited to how an adhesive is applied but include where it is applied. These two adhesives chemically react with tissues to form a strong bond. Therefore, it is not unexpected that when used near the nerves, there may be some undesired outcomes.[36] Such effects can be avoided by taking precautions, such as the use of surgical lubricants.[37] The effects of the individual components of surgical adhesive have also been seen with fibrin-based adhesives. Most recently, the effect of tranexamic acid, an antifibrinolytic agent, has been noted.[38] Similarly, surgeons have to consider the rate of growth of the patient or tissue (ie, use in children) and the rate of degradation of the adhesive being applied,[39] although there appear to be differences in the interpretation of the outcome in very similar models.[40]

One should also be reminded that surgical adhesives are not a replacement for good surgical technique. An adequate number of staples and suture should be placed to secure an anastomosis. This is important because all surgical sealants and adhesives are applied as liquids. This presents the opportunity for the adhesive to enter the lumen of a vessel if the repair is not adequate. Such a possibility has been reported during in vitro studies.[41] This finding is not unique and has been reported independently for other glues.[13,42]

The IFU for BioGlue is more detailed with respect to the application of the product, such as not using the product intravascularly; avoiding exposing nerves to it; avoiding repeat exposure of the same patient to it; drying the surgical field; covering the surrounding tissue; not compressing the area of application; use of dilators, balloon catheters, or surgical sponges to closely approximate the dissected layers of the aorta; and applying only a thin layer of BioGlue to the targeted repair sites.

CONCLUSIONS

The last decade has experienced a proliferation of surgical adhesives for a multitude of surgical specialties. As seen above and elsewhere in this book, all of these are very effective tools, differing in their adhesive strength, polymerization time, resorbtion time, and resorbtion pathways. All of these different properties provide today's surgeon with a palette of surgical adhesives from which to choose. As their use becomes more widespread, the use of two (or more) different surgical adhesives for different stages of surgery on the same patient (eg, for vascular closure and skin closure) is becoming a reality. The next frontier will be the use of surgical adhesives in robotic surgery.

REFERENCES

1. Saltz R, Toriumi DM, editors. Tissue glues in cosmetic surgery. St. Louis (MO): Quality Medical Publishing; 2004.

2. Braunwald NS, Tatooles CJ. Use of a cross linked gelatin tissue adhesive to control hemorrhage from liver and kidney. Surg Forum 1965;16:345–6.

3. Braunwald NS, Gay W, Tatooles CJ. Evaluation of crosslinked gelatin as a tissue adhesive and hemostatic agent: an experimental study. Surgery 1966;59:1024–30.

4. Bachet J, Gigou F, Laurian C, et al. Four year clinical experience with the gelatin-resorcine-formol biological glue in aortic dissection. J Thorac Cardiovasc Surg 1982;83:212–7.

5. Bachet J, Goudot B, Teodori G, et al. Surgery of type A acute aortic dissection with gelatine-resorcine-formol biological glue: a twelve-year experience. J Cardiovasc Surg (Torino) 1990;31:263–73.

6. Bachet J, Goudot B, Dreyfus G, et al. The proper use of glue: a 20 year experience with the GRF glue in aortic dissection. J Card Surg 1997;12:243–55.

7. Ennker IC, Ennker J, Schoon D, et al. Formaldehyde-free collagen glue in experimental lung gluing. Ann Thorac Surg 1994;57:1622–7.

8. Wertzel H, Wagner B, Stricker A, et al. Experimental gluing of lung parenchyma in rats. Thorac Cardiovasc Surg 1997;45:83–7.

9. Bellotto F, Johnson RG, Weintraub RM, et al. Pneumostasis of injured lung in rabbits with gelatin-resorcinol formaldehyde-glutaraldehyde tissue adhesive. Surg Gynecol Obstet 1992;174:221–4.

10. Nomori H, Horio H. Gelatin-resorcinol-formaldehyde-glutaraldehyde glue-spread stapler prevents air leakage from the lung [published erratum appears in Ann Thorac Surg 1997;64:892]. Ann Thorac Surg 1997;63:352–5.

11. Tanaka K, Takamoto S, Ohtsuka T, et al. Application of AdvaSeal for acute aortic dissection: experimental study. Ann Thorac Surg 1999;68:1308–12; discussion 1312–3.

12. Macchiarini P, Wain J, Almy S, Dartevelle P. Experimental and clinical evaluation of a new synthetic, absorbable sealant to reduce air leaks in thoracic operations. J Thorac Cardiovasc Surg 1999;117:751–8.

13. Hill A, Estridge TD, Maroney M, et al. Treatment of suture line bleeding with a novel synthetic surgical sealant in a canine iliac PTFE graft model. J Biomed Mater Res 2001;58:308–12.

14. Wallace DG, Cruise GM, Rhee WM, et al. A tissue sealant based on reactive multifunctional polyethylene glycol. J Biomed Mater Res 2001;58:545–55.

15. US Food and Drug Administration. Cohesion Technologies' CoSeal surgical sealant review memorandum by Jennifer L. Goode August 8, 2001. Available at: http://www.fda.gov/ohrms/dockets/ac/01/briefing/3790b2_05_fda.pdf (accessed Dec 12, 2003).

16. Gundry SR, Black K, Izutani H. Sutureless coronary artery bypass with biologic glued anastomoses: preliminary in vivo and in vitro results. J Thorac Cardiovasc Surg. 2000;120:473–7.

17. Hewitt CW, Marra SW, Kann BR, et al. BioGlue surgical adhesive for thoracic aortic repair during coagulopathy: efficacy and histopathology. Ann Thorac Surg 2001;71:1609–12.

18. Erasmi AW, Sievers HH, Wolschlager C. Inflammatory response after BioGlue application. Ann Thorac Surg 2002;73:1025–6.

19. Glickman M, Gheissari A, Money S, et al. A polymeric sealant inhibits anastomotic suture hole bleeding more rapidly than Gelfoam/thrombin: results of a randomized controlled trial. Arch Surg 2002;137:326–31; discussion 332.

20. US Food and Drug Administration. Instructions for use, CoSeal Surgical Sealant. Available at: http://www.fda.gov/ohrms/dockets/ac/01/briefing/3790b2_03_cohesion.pdf (accessed Dec 16, 2003).

21. Eddy AC, Capps SB, Chi E, et al. The effects of BioGlue Surgical Adhesive in the surgical repair of aortic dissection in sheep. Presented at the 12th Annual Meeting of theEuropean Association for Cardio-Thoracic Surgery; 1998 Sept 20–23; Brussels, Belgium.

22. Coselli JS, Bavaria JE, Fehrenbacher J, et al. Prospective randomized study of a protein-based tissue adhesive used as a hemostatic and structural adjunct in cardiac and vascular anastomotic repair procedures. J Am Coll Surg 2003;197:243–52; discussion 252–3.

23. US Food and Drug Administration. Available at: http://www.fda.gov/cdrh/pma/pmamar03.html (accessed Dec 12, 2003).

24. Hendrikx M, Mees U, Hill AC, et al. Evaluation of a novel synthetic sealant for inhibition of cardiac adhesions and clinical experience in cardiac surgery procedures. Heart Surg Forum 2001;4:204–9; discussion 210.

25. Konertz WF, Kostelka M, Mohr FW, et al. Reducing the incidence and severity of pericardial adhesions with a sprayable polymeric matrix. Ann Thorac Surg 2003;76:1270–74; discussion 1274.

26. Alamanni F, Fumero A, Parolari A, et al. Sutureless double-patch-and-glue technique for repair of subacute left ventricular wall rupture after myocardial infarction. J Thorac Cardiovasc Surg. 2001;122:836–7.

27. Coselli JS, LeMaire SA, Köksoy C. Thoracic aortic anastomoses. Oper Techn Thorac Cardiovasc Surg 2000;5:259–76.

28. Küçükaksu DS, Akgül A, Çagli K, Tasdemir O. Beneficial effect of BioGlue surgical adhesive in repair of iatrogenic aortic dissection. Tex Heart Inst J 2000;27:307–8.

29. Raanani E, Latter D, Errett LE, et al. Use of "BioGlue" in aortic surgical repair. Ann Thorac Surg 2001;72:638–40.

30. Fink D, Klein JJ, Kang H, Ergin A. Application of biological glue in repair of intracardiac structural defects. Ann Thorac Surg 2004;77:506–11.

31. Herget GW, Kassa M, Riede UN, et al. Experimental use of an albumin-glutaraldehyde tissue adhesive for sealing pulmonary parenchyma and bronchial anastomoses. Eur J Cardiothorac Surg 2001;19(1):4–9.

32. Lai MH, Storey DW, Hughes CF. Repair of major airway injury using albumin-glutaraldehyde glue. Aust N Z J Surg 2001;71: 555–6.

33. Potaris K, Mihos P, Gakidis I. Experience with an albumin glutaraldehyde tissue adhesive in sealing air leaks after bullectomy. Heart Surg Forum 2003;6:429–33.

34. Lin J, Iannettoni MD. Closure of bronchopleural fistulas using albumin-glutaraldehyde tissue adhesive. Ann Thorac Surg. 2004;74:326–8.

35. Kumar A, Maartens NF, Kaye AH. Evaluation of the use of BioGlue® in neurosurgical procedures. J Clin Neurosci 2003;10:661–4.

36. LeMaire SA, Schmittling ZC, Ündar A, et al. A new surgical adhesive (BioGlue) causes acute phrenic nerve injury and diaphragmatic paralysis. Presented at the 34th Annual Meeting of the Association for Academic Surgery; 2000 Nov 2–4; Tampa, FL.

37. LeMaire SA, Conklin LD, Schmittling ZC, et al. Chlorhexidine gluconate gel protects exposed nerves during the application of BioGlue surgical adhesive. Presented at the Association for Academic Surgery 35th Annual Meeting; 2001 Nov 5–17; Milwaukee, WI.

38. US Food and Drug Administration. Labeling information for Crosseal™ fibrin sealant (human). Available at: http://www.fda.gov/cber/label/fibomri032103LB.pdf (accessed Dec 16, 2003).

39. LeMaire SA, Schmittling ZC, Coselli JS, et al. BioGlue surgical adhesive impairs aortic growth and causes anastomotic strictures. Ann Thorac Surg. 2002;73:1500–5; discussion 1506.

40. Glock Y, Roux D, Leobon B, et al. Experimental technique of aorto-prosthetic anastomoses by gluing (BioGlue® CryoLife). Presented at the Laparoscopic Aortoiliac Surgery for Occlusive Disease and Aneurysms Symposium. 2000 Jan 28; Marseilles, France.

41. LeMaire SA, Won T, Conklin LD, et al. Expanded polytetrafluoroethylene (ePTFE) suture does not eliminate the risk of adhesive leakage in ePTFE grafts. Presented at the Tissue Sealants and Adhesives Workshop; 2003 Sept 20–21; Orlando, FL.

42. Tonner PH, Scholz J. Possible lung embolism following embolization of a hemangioma with fibrin glue. Anaesthesist 1994;43:614–7.

43. Barrows TH, Lewis TW, Truong MT, inventors; Minnesota Mining and Manufacturing Company, assignee. Adhesive sealant composition. US patent 5,583,114. 1996 Dec 10.

44. Wilkie J, Rolke J, Burzio L, et al. Methods and compositions for sealing tissue leaks. US patent application US 2002/0022588. 2002 Feb 21.

45. Allen MS, Wood DE, Harpole DH, et al. Prospective randomized study evaluating a biodegradable polymeric sealant for sealing intraoperative air leaks that occur during pulmonary resection. Presented at the 39th Annual Meeting of the Society for Thoracic Surgeons; 2003 Jan 31–Feb 2; San Diego, CA.

6 Bone Cements

Jennifer L. Maw, MD, FRCS

History and Background

The use of cements as fixation devices dates back to the mid-twentienth century. They were first used in dentistry but were truly popularized by an innovative surgeon, Sir John Charnley. He revolutionized the care of persons with arthritic hips and knees by introducing joint replacement surgery using polymethylmethacrylate, commonly known as "bone cement," to fixate the prosthesis. Based on his founding principles, over 100,000 hip replacement surgeries are performed each year in the United States. There have been many improvements in technique, methods, and materials for cement fixation since the original bone cement was found to eventually break down.

The search for a moldable material to augment and integrate bone repair has continued for many decades. Bone grafting procedures are common; an estimated 500,000 to 600,000 are performed annually in the United States.[1] Autogenous bone is the superior graft because it is osteogenic (contains viable cells), osteoinductive (contains growth factors), and osteoconductive (has a matrix for new bone formation to grow through). It is nonimmunogenic and nonpathogenic when handled in a sterile environment. The disadvantages of autogenous bone grafting include the expense of the harvesting procedure in prolonged operating room time and recovery time, the morbidity of the donor site, and the degree of resorption over long-term follow-up. The latter can result in a cosmetic deformity requiring secondary corrective procedures.

Bone cements and bone graft substitutes are becoming more popular as experience with these products grows. It would be impossible in this chapter to review and discuss the numerous materials labeled and marketed as cements and bone substitutes and to further review their innumerable reported clinical uses. Instead, this chapter provides an overview of bone graft substitutes and focuses on bone cements. The field is very dynamic, and at the time of writing, many new products are on the horizon. I urge the reader to carefully review the US Food and Drug Administration (FDA) Web site to keep apprised of the current status of approved indications for particular products (<http://www.fda.gov/cdrh/>).

ALLOGRAFTS AND XENOGRAFTS

Allografts are transplants from other human beings or cadavers and can be frozen or freeze-dried, but bone bank material is limited in quantity compared with the volume required. Allografts have less strength and osteogenic potential than autografts and carry the potential risk of infectious transmission, such as hepatitis or human immunodeficiency virus (HIV).

Many engineered allografts have been approved by the FDA, and many are in development.[2] They eliminate the problem of limited quantity but are not without problems. Demineralized bone matrix (DBM) grafts can be produced as gels, flexible sheets, or putty and consist of a collagenous matrix that can be remineralized in the patient's body; they show osteoinductive properties[3] but do not give any structural support. Several products are available, approved for nonunion, delayed, and potentially delayed unions. Grafton DBM (Osteotech Inc., Eatontown, NJ) is available as a gel, putty, or semi-rigid product. Osteofil (Sofamor Danek Group, Inc., Memphis, TN) contains 24% DBM and 17% porcine gelatin in an aqueous solution that can flow through a syringe. Opteform (Exactech, Inc, Gainsville, FL) contains Osteofil and corticocancellous human bone chips in a moldable, putty form. It is thought to be more osteoinductive than DBM alone and is approved for acetabulum, calcaneous, and tibial plateau reconstruction. Intergro (Interpore Cross International, Irvine, CA) DBM putty combines DBM with a lecithin to form a putty for easy handling and moldability. Extensive animal data exist in these products, but there is limited evidence from human trials that they provide significant concentrations of BMP to be osseoinductive. They are derived from cadaveric bone, with potential immunogenic and pathogenic concerns.

The available xenografts are mostly bovine, with the same advantages and disadvantages as allografts but with the added concerns of potential immunogenic reactions and prion infection. Collagraft (Zimmer, Inc, Warsaw, IN) was approved by the FDA in 1993 and is available as a paste or strips. It is a mixture of granules containing 65% hydroxyapatite (HA), 35% tricalcium phosphate, and type I bovine collagen. It is mixed with aspirated autologous bone marrow. It has been used for diaphyseal and metaphyseal defects[4–6] but provides no structural support and is used in conjunction with internal fixation. It is FDA approved for bone defects of the spine, extremities, and pelvis.

SYNTHETIC BONE GRAFT SUBSTITUTES

Coral-Based Products

Coral-based products are derived from converting reef-building marine corals into coralline HA through a hydrothermal chemical exchange reaction.[7] During the reaction, all organic material is removed, but its architecture is preserved. The matrix is composed of calcium carbonate covered by a thin layer of HA. Coralline HA has been used as a bone graft substitute for more than 20 years.[7–10] Initial products resorbed slowly and were considered relatively permanent implants. New bone forms on the surface of the implant and is distributed throughout the porous structure. These products can be mixed with autograft or used alone. Disadvantages include low tensile strength and brittleness.

Pro-Osteon (Interpore Cross International, Irvine, CA) was approved by the FDA in 1992 for a filler of acute, traumatic metaphyseal bone defects. It is made from the Porites marine coral as its porous microstructure is structurally similar to cancellous bone. Pro-Osteon-200 is FDA approved for craniofacial, maxillofacial, and periodontal defects and alveolar ridge augmentation. Pro-Osteon 500, made from Goniopora coral, has a larger pore size and is approved for metaphyseal fracture defects, long bone cysts, and tumor defects in conjunction with rigid internal fixation and spinal fusions. Pro-Osteon R is a more resorbable coralline product with a layer of HA on its surface. These products are osteoconductive and participate in the osteogenic and osteoinductive processes. All research and clinical applications confirm it to be an osteoconductive implant.[1] They have been successfully used in the treatment of fractures of the tibial plateau, radius, and spine.[11–13]

Acceptance by the orthopedic community is far from complete, with concerns regarding the mechanism and time course of resorption and its visibility on a radiograph for long periods of time. Despite its resemblance to bone, osteoclastic resorption has not been shown, and the potential for true remodeling is likely limited.[2]

Calcium Sulfate Substitutes

Calcium sulfate, or plaster of Paris, has been used as a bone void filler for over a century, with inconsistent findings. This may have been secondary to the variable quality and presence of contaminating trace elements. Medical grade products are now available. Given that calcium sulfate was marketed in the United States before the current FDA approval process, no clinical trial data were required for FDA clearance in 1996. Osteoset (Wright Medical, Arlington, TN) is supplied in 3 and 4.8 mm hard pellets, and Bone Plast (Interpore Cross International) is a moldable form of calcium sulfate. Newer products include Stimulan (Encore, Austin, TX), a mixture of DBM and calcium sulfate, and Allomatrix (Wright Medical), a combination of calcium and DBM.

Calcium sulfate has been shown to be an effective osteoconductive bone graft substitute. The mechanism of action is unknown, but it allows osseous ingrowth to occur in bone defects while preventing ingrowth of soft tissue. Animal research has demonstrated that osteoblasts attach to the surface of the pellets, whereas osteoclasts can resorb it.[14] It is resorbed variably by 6 to 8 weeks. It has been used for bone defects from trauma and benign bone tumor resections, revision hip and knee surgery, and spinal arthodeses.[15,16] The use of rigid fixation is required because calcium sulfate does not provide structural support.

Bioactive Glass

Bioglass (US BIOmaterials Corporation, Alachua, FL) is an FDA-approved silica product for periodontal indications. It is a synthetic bone graft substitute composed of silicon, sodium, calcium, and phosphorous oxides. The product is porous, with bead sizes ranging from 90 to 710 μm. The glass beads bond to collagen, fibrin, and growth factors, forming a matrix at the implant site. It is postulated that the slow release of silicon produces an autocrine response with enhancement of osteoblastic activity. Osteogenic cells infiltrate the material and make new bone. It has proven useful for dental, oral, and maxillofacial surgery[17–20] and ossicular chain reconstruction[21–23] and is being investigated for mastoid reconstruction.[24] Its popularity in orthopedics has been limited owing to its limited structural support. It is approved in Europe for orthopedic indications under the name NovaBone.

Bone Cements

Bone cements have been used as moldable, stable materials to eliminate the morbidity of autografts and the concerns of allografts and xenografts. The ideal material still elludes us but would be inexpensive, easy to use, and biocompatible; would allow replacement by host bone; and would be associated with a low rate of infection.

Methylmethacrylate

Methylmethacrylate is a polymethacrylate cement made by combining methylmethacrylate monomer liquid with a methylmethacrylate-styrene copolymer powder. It is the most common "bone cement" and has the longest history of use. It is a cost-effective and inert material that can be molded to a predictable shape. Problems include the exothermic reaction, which can generate significant temperatures and be injurious to tissues, and the need for rigid fixation to prevent it from coming loose over time. The carcinogenic potential to humans is also unknown but is unlikely, given the long experience with its use. Its biocompatibility has also been questioned because there is no tissue ingrowth into the implant. Despite this, it remains the most frequently used alloplastic material for reconstruction worldwide.[25]

An FDA warning has been issued regarding its use when treating compression fractures of the spine. The report outlines complications involving leakage causing local nerve root irritation and compression, as well as systemic complications, such as pulmonary embolism and cardiac failure. The warning specifically mentions that it is inappropriate to use it for load-bearing indications (see <http://www.fda.gov/cdrh/safety/bonecement.html>).

Polycarboxylate Cements

Early varieties of these cements have been used in dentistry as leuting materials since the 1970s. These cements bond strongly to bone, and a long-term stability of greater than 50 years has been shown. These cements are not osseoinductive but are considered permanent.

Glass ionomeric cements are made from an aluminum silicate powder and a polyalkenoic liquid of polycarboxylates. The cement can be shaped somewhat prior to hardening. Although isothermic, aluminum and calcium ions are released and are soluble during the chemical reaction, and a dry environment must be achieved during the setting time of 10 to 20 minutes. Once hardened, the cement is thought to no longer be sensitive to surrounding fluids. Ionomeric cements have been used for ossicular chain reconstruction (Figures 6–1 and 6–2),[26–31] external auditory canal reconstruction,[32,33] cochlear implant fixation,[34] and middle ear implantable device coupling[35] and have proven useful for tegmen reconstruction[27] and mastoid obliteration.[27,28,36–38] Their use in neurotology and skull base surgery has been limited because of aluminum toxicity. Ionocap was withdrawn from the European market after several fatalities occurred from aluminum toxicity when the material was in contact with cerebrospinal fluid. In the United States, only SerenoCem (Corinthian Surgical Ltd, Corinthian Surgical Ltd, Harrowgate, N Yorkshire, UK) is currently available.

Calcium Phosphate Cements

Calcium phosphate cements (CPCs) were first discovered by Brown and Chow in the mid-1980s and became popular and effective in the dental and orthopedic fields. CPCs contain low-temperature calcium phosphate, and the end product of the setting reaction of CPC is always a low-temperature calcium phosphate. CPCs are nonceramic, low-temperature apatites that are moldable, closely resemble the mineral phase of bone, and chemically bond to the host bone. They are made of an aqueous solution and of one or several calcium phosphates. They do not harden through a polymerization reaction, and minimal heat is released. They have a low tensile strength and are used in non–load-bearing applications. They are rapidly emerging as preferred materials for reconstruction of the craniofacial skeleton.

Most products have a porosity of around 50 vol%, with a pore size of close to 1 µm. The small pore size is not compatible with fast ingrowth of bone, and the CPC degrades layer by layer. They are thought to potentially be bioactive in that they may allow bioresorption and osteoconductivity or be resorbed and replaced progressively by newly formed host bone.[39–41]

HA cement (BoneSource, Stryker-Leibinger Corp., Kalamazoo, MI), Dahllite cement (Norian CRS, Norian, Cupertino, CA), and the Mimix HA bone replacement system (Biomet/W. Lorenz Surgical,

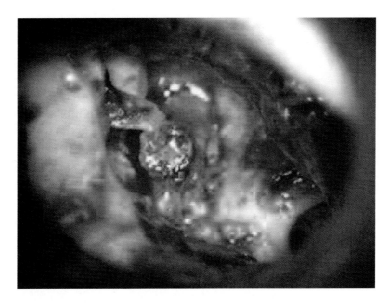

FIGURE 6-1 Ossicular chain incus erosion.

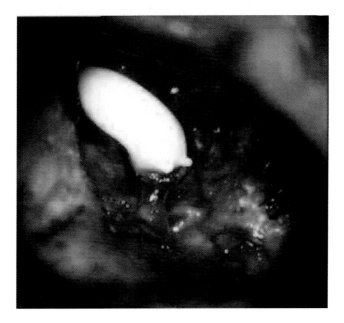

FIGURE 6-2 Ossicular chain repair with ionomeric cement.

Jacksonville, FL) are FDA approved materials for skull base recon-struction. Other new HA cements include Alpha-BSM (ETEX Cor-poration) and Biopex (Mitsubishi Materials Incorporated, Tokyo, Japan).

Bone Source was the first CPC to become widely used in craniofacial surgery.[42] It is a combination of tetracalcium phosphate and dicalcium phosphate that is mixed with a sodium phosphate solution. It forms a paste that sets in 20 minutes and hardens in 24 hours. It has proven useful for skull base reconstruction and cerebrospinal fluid leak repair of the lateral and anterior skull base[43–49] and is also used for reconstruction of frontal bone fractures.[50] It has also been found effective for ossicular chain reconstruction in erosion of the incudostapedial joint.[51] Bone Source has also been used in repair of traumatic metaphyseal bone voids of type I fractures.[52]

Norian is a carbonated calcium phosphate paste. It is composed of calcium phosphate and calcium carbonate, which are mixed with sodium phosphate and form Dahllite, a carbonated apatite. It is available as an injectable paste (Norian CRS) or moldable putty (Fast Set Putty) that sets in 10 or 6 minutes, respectively, and hardens over 24 hours. It is FDA approved for cranial reconstruction of defects less than 25 cm^2, Colles' fracture repair, tibial plateau, and calcaneous uses (Figure 6–3). It has proven effective in the repair of distal radius fractures in a prospective, randomized, multicenter trial, leading to accelerated rehabilitation versus controls in which no CRS was used.[53] Dahllite has also been used as an adjunct in the repair of femoral neck fractures[54] and facial fractures.[55] It has been investigated for ossicular chain reconstruction in an animal model.[56]

Mimix is formed by tetracalcium and tricalcium phosphate. It is supplied as a white powder that is mixed with citric acid to form a paste that hardens quickly but requires a dry and blood-free surgical site. It has been used for cranioplasty[57] and external auditory canal wall reconstruction in a gerbil model.[58]

CPCs are marketed as being bioactive in that they may allow bioresorption and osteoinduction or be resorbed and replaced progressively by newly formed host bone while maintaining their shape and volume. They may initiate osteogenesis or promote osteoconduction when placed in direct contact with host bone.[59] The process is thought to be cell-mediated resorption by osteoclasts followed by new bone formation by osteoblasts. There is animal evidence of this bioactivity in long bones,[60] but there is controversy as to the extent to which this occurs in the skull.[61] This process is thought to occur over years, depending on metabolic rate and loading. With little to no loading in the cranium, remodeling is thought to occur slowly.

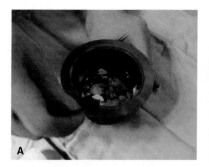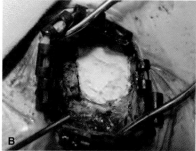

■ FIGURE 6-3   Cement preparation (*A*) and reconstruction (*B*) of the sigmoid skull base using Dahllite cement.

Although CPCs seem to be biocompatible and have been used in children,[62,63] osteoinduction has not been demonstrated. Studies have demonstrated a lack of bone replacement in animal models when used for dental extractions[64] and in the rabbit calvarium.[65] It should be noted that the majority of the work in this field has been industry sponsored. The industry claims of bone replacement have not been substantiated in the peer-reviewed literature.[66]

Early results seem promising, but long-term follow-up studies have not been so enthusiastic. Significant complications have been reported in the use of HA cement for craniofacial contour refinements[67] and calvarial reconstruction,[25] frontal bone reconstruction,[68] and pediatric craniofacial and skull base surgery.[69] Thinning and erosion of the skin over the implant, the presence of infection, and extrusion of the material can make secondary procedures difficult and compound the reconstructive problem.

Significant failures and complications occurred with both Dahllite and HA cement for mastoid obliteration and external auditory canal wall reconstruction (Figure 6–4).[70,71] I experienced good initial results, but long-term follow-up revealed breakdown of the cement, extrusion, and infection, with secondary procedures required for removal and reconstruction. More long-term studies are required to characterize the long-term efficacy and safety of CPCs.

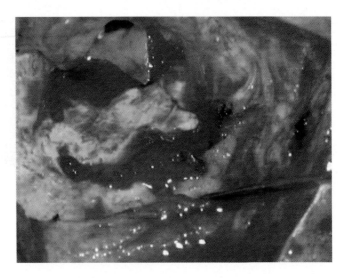

■ FIGURE 6-4   Extrusion of Dahllite cement when used for mastoid obliteration.

CONCLUSION

Synthetic bone graft substitutes and bone cements are increasing in popularity for bone grafting procedures. Bodies of literature exist that strongly support their use in various fields, whereas other authors have concerns. Despite two decades of experience with various products, there is a paucity of well-designed clinical trials showing benefit or cost-effectiveness. The degree to which these products are osteoconductive varies in the peer-reviewed literature, and standardized testing is lacking. Compounds address some of the disadvantages of autogenous bone grafting because they are unlimited in supply, sterile, and easy to use. They are not without disadvantages because they are costly, result in variable bone resorption and replacement, and have potential adverse effects on normal bone remodeling. There is a lack of clinical efficacy studies for many of their potential indications.

Future materials will likely improve with the addition of pharmaceuticals and bone growth hormones, and these products will likely show benefit as carriers of the substrates to accelerate healing. It is hoped that future studies will delineate the clinical contraindications that have led to failure and concern.

Finally, with the speed at which this field is changing and new innovations are occurring, the surgeon is once again urged to keep updated of FDA-approved uses and advisories, to review the literature prior to use, to report complications to the FDA, and to publish both favorable and unfavorable findings in the literature.

REFERENCES

1. Bucholz RW. Nonallograft osteoconductive bone graft substitutes. Clin Orthop 2002;395:44–52.

2. Ladd AL, Pliam NB. The role of bone graft and alternatives in unstable distal radius fracture treatment. Orthop Clin North Am 2001;32:337–51, ix.

3. Urist MR, Silverman BF, Buring K, et al. The bone induction principle. Clin Orthop 1967;53:243–83.

4. Chapman MW, Bucholz R, Cornell C. Treatment of acute fractures with a collagen-calcium phosphate graft material. A randomized clinical trial. J Bone Joint Surg Am 1997;79:495–502.

5. Moore DC, Chapman MW, Manske D. The evaluation of a biphasic calcium phosphate ceramic for use in grafting long-bone diaphyseal defects. J Orthop Res 1987;5:356–65.

6. Grundel RE, Chapman MW, Yee T, Moore DC. Autogeneic bone marrow and porous biphasic calcium phosphate ceramic for segmental bone defects in the canine ulna. Clin Orthop 1991;266:244–58.

7. Roy DM, Linnehan SK. Hydroxyapatite formed from coral skeletal carbonate by hydrothermal exchange. Nature 1974;247:220–2.

8. Chiroff RT, White EW, Weber KN, Roy DM. Tissue ingrowth of Replamineform implants. J Biomed Mater Res 1975;9:29–45.

9. Guillemin G, Patat JL, Fournie J, Chetail M. The use of coral as a bone graft substitute. J Biomed Mater Res 1987;21:557–67.

10. Sartoris DJ, Gershuni DH, Akeson WH, et al. Coralline hydroxyapatite bone graft substitutes: preliminary report of radiographic evaluation. Radiology 1986;159:133–7.

11. Bucholz RW, Carlton A, Holmes R. Interporous hydroxyapatite as a bone graft substitute in tibial plateau fractures. Clin Orthop 1989;240:53–62.

12. Wolfe SW, Pike L, Slade JF III, Katz LD. Augmentation of distal radius fracture fixation with coralline hydroxyapatite bone graft substitute. J Hand Surg [Am] 1999;24:816–27.

13. Thalgott JS, Giuffre JM, Klezl Z, Timlin M. Anterior lumbar interbody fusion with titanium mesh cages, coralline hydroxyapatite, and demineralized bone matrix as part of a circumferential fusion. Spine J 2002;2:63–9.

14. Sidqui M, Collin P, Vitte C, Forest N. Osteoblast adherence and resorption activity of isolated osteoclasts on calcium sulphate hemihydrate. Biomaterials 1995;16:1327–32.

15. Kelly CM, Wilkins RM, Gitelis S, et al. The use of a surgical grade calcium sulfate as a bone graft substitute: results of a multicenter trial. Clin Orthop 2001;382:42–50.

16. Gitelis S, Piasecki P, Turner T, et al. Use of a calcium sulfate-based bone graft substitute for benign bone lesions. Orthopedics 2001;24:162–6.

17. Lovelace TB, Mellonig JT, Meffert RM, et al. Clinical evaluation of bioactive glass in the treatment of periodontal osseous defects in humans. J Periodontol 1998;69:1027–35.

18. Low SB, King CJ, Krieger J. An evaluation of bioactive ceramic in the treatment of periodontal osseous defects. Int J Periodont Restor Dent 1997;17:358–67.

19. Shapoff CA, Alexander DC, Clark AE. Clinical use of a bioactive glass particulate in the treatment of human osseous defects. Compend Contin Educ Dent 1997;18:352–4, 356, 358.

20. Peltola M, Suonpaa J, Aitasalo K, et al. Obliteration of the frontal sinus cavity with bioactive glass. Head Neck 1998;20:315–9.

21. Rust KR, Singleton GT, Wilson J, Antonelli PJ. Bioglass middle ear prosthesis: long-term results. Am J Otol 1996;17:371–4.

22. Niparko JK, Kemink JL, Graham MD, Kartush JM. Bioactive glass ceramic in ossicular reconstruction: a preliminary report. Laryngoscope 1988;98(8 Pt 1):822–5.

23. Reck R, Storkel S, Meyer A. Bioactive glass-ceramics in middle ear surgery. An 8-year review. Ann N Y Acad Sci 1988;523:100–6.

24. Leatherman BD, Dornhoffer JL. Bioactive glass ceramic particles as an alternative for mastoid obliteration: results in an animal model. Otol Neurotol 2002;23:657–60; discussion 660.

25. Moreira-Gonzalez A, Jackson IT, Miyawaki T, et al. Clinical outcome in cranioplasty: critical review in long-term follow-up. J Craniofac Surg 2003;14:144–53.

26. Geyer G, Stadtgen A, Schwager K, Jonck L. Ionomeric cement implants in the middle ear of the baboon (*Papio ursinus*) as a primate model. Eur Arch Otorhinolaryngol 1998;255:402–9.

27. Kupperman D, Tange RA. Ionomeric cement in the human middle ear cavity: long-term results of 23 cases. Laryngoscope 2001;111:306–9.

28. Kupperman D, Tange RA. Long-term results of glass ionomer cement, Ionocem, in the middle ear of the rat. Acta Otorhinolaryngol Belg 1997;51:27–30.

29. McElveen JT Jr, Feghali JG, Barrs DM, et al. Ossiculoplasty with polymaleinate ionomeric prosthesis. Otolaryngol Head Neck Surg 1995;113:420–6.

30. McElveen JT Jr. Ossiculoplasty with polymaleinate ionomeric pros-theses. Otolaryngol Clin North Am 1994;27:777–84.

31. Chen DA, Arriaga MA. Technical refinements and precautions during ionomeric cement reconstruction of incus erosion during revision stapedectomy. Laryngoscope 2003;113:848–52.

32. McElveen JT Jr, Chung AT. Reversible canal wall down mastoidectomy for acquired cholesteatomas: preliminary results. Laryngoscope 2003;113:1027–33.

33. Geyer G, Helms J. Ionomer-based bone substitute in otologic surgery. Eur Arch Otorhinolaryngol 1993;250:253–6.

34. Muller J, Geyer G, Helms J. [Ionomer cement in cochlear implant surgery]. Laryngorhinootologie 1993;72:36–8.

35. Ko WH, Zhu WL, Kane M, Maniglia AJ. Engineering principles applied to implantable otologic devices. Otolaryngol Clin North Am 2001;34:299–314.

36. Velich N, Nemeth Z, Toth C, Szabo G. Long-term results with differ-ent bone substitutes used for sinus floor elevation. J Craniofac Surg 2004;15:38–41.

37. Hsu CC, Wang JW, Chen CE, Lin JW. Results of curettage and high-speed burring for chondroblastoma of the bone. Chang Gung Med J 2003;26:761–7.

38. Jahng TA, Fu TS, Cunningham BW, et al. Endoscopic instrumented posterolateral lumbar fusion with Healos and recombinant human growth/differentiation factor-5. Neurosurgery 2004;54:171–80; dis-cussion 180–1.

39. Friedman CD, Costantino PD, Jones K, et al. Hydroxyapatite cement. II. Obliteration and reconstruction of the cat frontal sinus. Arch Otolaryngol Head Neck Surg 1991;117:385–9.

40. Losee JE, Karmacharya J, Gannon FH, et al. Reconstruction of the immature craniofacial skeleton with a carbonated calcium phos-phate bone cement: interaction with bioresorbable mesh. J Cranio-fac Surg 2003;14:117–24.

41. Ma Y, Xu X, Zhou TK, et al. [Experimental study on bioglass appli-cation in extending alveolar bone crest in rabbit]. Shanghai Kou Qiang Yi Xue 2001;10:240–2.

42. Bifano CA, Edgin WA, Colleton C, et al. Preliminary evaluation of hydroxyapatite cement as an augmentation device in the edentulous atrophic canine mandible. Oral Surg Oral Med Oral Pathol Oral Radiol Endod 1998;85:512–6.

43. Arriaga MA, Chen DA. Hydroxyapatite cement cranioplasty in translabyrinthine acoustic neuroma surgery. Otolaryngol Head Neck Surg 2002;126:512–7.

44. Kveton JF, Friedman CD, Piepmeier JM, Costantino PD. Reconstruc-tion of suboccipital craniectomy defects with hydroxyapatite

cement: a preliminary report. Laryngoscope 1995;105:156–9.

45. Kveton JF, Goravalingappa R. Elimination of temporal bone cerebrospinal fluid otorrhea using hydroxyapatite cement. Laryngoscope 2000;110(10 Pt 1):1655–9.

46. Costantino PD, Hiltzik DH, Sen C, et al. Sphenoethmoid cerebrospinal fluid leak repair with hydroxyapatite cement. Arch Otolaryngol Head Neck Surg 2001;127:588–93.

47. Kamerer DB, Hirsch BE, Snyderman CH, et al. Hydroxyapatite cement: a new method for achieving watertight closure in transtemporal surgery. Am J Otol 1994;15:47–9.

48. Hartl A, Bitzan P, Wanivenhaus A, Kotz R. Faster integration of human allograft bone than of the bovine substitute Lubboc: non-randomized evaluation of 20 cases with benign tumors or tumor-like conditions. Acta Orthop Scand 2004;75:217–20.

49. Kubler A, Neugebauer J, Oh JH, et al. Growth and proliferation of human osteoblasts on different bone graft substitutes: an in vitro study. Implant Dent 2004;13:171–9.

50. Chen TM, Wang HJ, Chen SL, Lin FH. Reconstruction of post-traumatic frontal-bone depression using hydroxyapatite cement. Ann Plast Surg 2004;52:303–8; discussion 309.

51. Babu S, Seidman MD. Ossicular reconstruction using bone cement. Otol Neurotol 2004;25:98–101.

52. Dickson KF, Friedman J, Buchholz JG, Flandry FD. The use of BoneSource hydroxyapatite cement for traumatic metaphyseal bone void filling. J Trauma 2002;53:1103–8.

53. Cassidy C, Jupiter JB, Cohen M, et al. Norian SRS cement compared with conventional fixation in distal radial fractures. A randomized study. J Bone Joint Surg Am 2003;85-A:2127–37.

54. Goodman SB, Bauer TW, Carter D, et al. Norian SRS cement augmentation in hip fracture treatment. Laboratory and initial clinical results. Clin Orthop 1998;348:42–50.

55. Wolff KD, Swaid S, Nolte D, et al. Degradable injectable bone cement in maxillofacial surgery: indications and clinical experience in 27 patients. J Craniomaxillofac Surg 2004;32:71–9.

56. Hoffmann KK, Kuhn JJ, Strasnick B. Bone cements as adjuvant techniques for ossicular chain reconstruction. Otol Neurotol 2003;24:24–8.

57. Moreira-Gonzalez A, Jackson IT, Miyawaki T, et al. Clinical outcome in cranioplasty: critical review in long-term follow-up. J Craniofac Surg 2003;14:144–53.

58. Dornhoffer J, Simmons O. Canal wall reconstruction with Mimix hydroxyapatite cement: results in an animal model and case study. Laryngoscope 2003;113:2123–8.

59. Stelnicki EJ, Ousterhout DK. Hydroxyapatite paste (BoneSource) used as an onlay implant for supraorbital and malar augmentation. J

Craniofac Surg 1997;8:367–72.

60. Frankenburg EP, Goldstein SA, Bauer TW, et al. Biomechanical and histological evaluation of a calcium phosphate cement. J Bone Joint Surg Am 1998;80:1112–24.

61. Clokie CM, Moghadam H, Jackson MT, Sandor GK. Closure of critical sized defects with allogenic and alloplastic bone substitutes. J Craniofac Surg 2002;13:111–21; discussion 122–3.

62. Baker SB, Weinzweig J, Kirschner RE, Bartlett SP. Applications of a new carbonated calcium phosphate bone cement: early experience in pediatric and adult craniofacial reconstruction. Plast Reconstr Surg 2002;109:1789–96.

63. Burstein FD, Cohen SR, Hudgins R, Boydston W. The use of porous granular hydroxyapatite in secondary orbitocranial reconstruction. Plast Reconstr Surg 1997;100:869–74.

64. Indovina A Jr, Block MS. Comparison of 3 bone substitutes in canine extraction sites. J Oral Maxillofac Surg 2002;60:53–8.

65. Moghadam HG, Sandor GK, Holmes HH, Clokie CM. Histomorphometric evaluation of bone regeneration using allogeneic and alloplastic bone substitutes. J Oral Maxillofac Surg 2004;62:202–13.

66. Schmitz JP, Hollinger JO, Milam SB. Reconstruction of bone using calcium phosphate bone cements: a critical review. J Oral Maxillofac Surg 1999;57:1122–6.

67. Jackson IT, Yavuzer R. Hydroxyapatite cement: an alternative for craniofacial skeletal contour refinements. Br J Plast Surg 2000;53:24–9.

68. Maniker A, Cantrell S, Vaicys C. Failure of hydroxyapatite cement to set in repair of a cranial defect: case report. Neurosurgery 1998;43:953–4; discussion 955.

69. Matic D, Phillips JH. A contraindication for the use of hydroxyapatite cement in the pediatric population. Plast Reconstr Surg 2002;110:1–5.

70. Mahendran S, Yung MW. Mastoid obliteration with hydroxyapatite cement: the Ipswich experience. Otol Neurotol 2004;25:19–21.

71. Maw JL. Mastoid obliteration with hydroxyapatite cement [abstract]. Otol Neurotol 2004;24:529–30.

7 US Food and Drug Administration Perspective on the Regulation of Medical Device Tissue Adhesives

CDR Stephen P. Rhodes, USPHS

The US Food and Drug Administration (FDA) is the federal agency responsible for ensuring that medical devices are safe and effective. The FDA ensures that these products are honestly, accurately, and informatively represented to the public. The FDA is also responsible for advancing public health by helping to speed innovations that make devices more effective, safer, and more affordable and by helping the public obtain the accurate, science-based information that it needs to use devices to improve health. The FDA evaluates and approves or clears new medical products for the marketplace, inspects manufacturing facilities before and during commercial distribution, and takes corrective action to remove products from commerce when they are unsafe, ineffective, misbranded, or adulterated. The burden of proof with regard to the product's safety and effectiveness is the responsibility of the manufacturer. The premarket review of all products is based on the manufacturer's stated intended use of each product and the information submitted.

To accomplish its mission over the wide range of products in its regulatory purview, the FDA has six centers, each staffed with the scientific and regulatory expertise to evaluate the products in the center's jurisdiction. The Center for Devices and Radiological Health (CDRH) is responsible for the regulation of medical devices and radiation-emitting products in the United States. The CDRH seeks to protect public health by ensuring reasonable assurance of the safety and effectiveness of medical devices and by eliminating unnecessary human exposure to radiation emitted from electronic products. An important portion of the products that CDRH regulates arises from new technologic achievements and innovations. An example of a new technologic innovation is the tissue adhesive products developed through engineering and biologic principles for use in a wide range of surgical interventions.

PREMARKET REVIEW OF MEDICAL DEVICES

The FDA regulates the development, testing, production, and distribution of medical devices. Prior to 1976, the FDA had the authority to restrict the marketing of unsafe or ineffective devices through limited provisions in the federal Food, Drug, and Cosmetic Act of 1938 and through judicial extensions. The act was amended under provisions of the Medical Device Amendments of 1976, which greatly expanded the role of the FDA in the regulation of medical devices. The amendments included a broad definition of a device, provisions for actions against violative products, a tiered system of regulation, participation of outside experts (advisory panels), an expanded scope of evidence for effectiveness claims, limitations on trade secret information, and extensive procedural safeguards.

The amendments directed the FDA to classify all devices into one of three classes, depending on the amount of regulation required to ensure reasonable assurance of safety and effectiveness. For class I devices, general controls are sufficient to ensure safety and efficacy. General controls include provisions that relate to adulteration; misbranding; device registration and listing; premarket notification; banned devices; notification, including repair, replacement, or refund; records and reports; restricted devices; and good manufacturing practices. Manual surgical instruments, such as blades and trocars, are class I devices. Most class I devices are now exempt from premarket notification. Devices are placed in class II if general controls are insufficient to ensure safety and effectiveness. For class II devices, there is sufficient information to establish "special controls," which may include guidance documents, performance standards, or device tracking to provide assurance. An example of a class II device is an absorbable suture. Class III devices are those for which insufficient information exists to ensure safety and effectiveness solely through general or special controls. An example of a class III device is a cyanoacrylate neurologic embolization device that polymerizes in situ.

Each person who wants to market class I and II and some class III devices intended for human use in the United States must submit a premarket notification [510(k)] to the FDA at least 90 days before marketing unless the device is exempt from 510(k) requirements. A 510(k) is a premarketing submission made to the FDA to demonstrate that the device to be marketed is as safe and effective, that is, substantially equivalent to, a marketed device that is not subject to premarket approval (PMA). Applicants must compare their 510(k) device to one or more similar devices currently on the US market and make and support their substantial equivalency claims.

PMA is the FDA process of scientific and regulatory review to evaluate the safety and effectiveness of class III medical devices. Class III devices are those that support or sustain human life, are of substantial importance in preventing impairment of human health, or present a potential, unreasonable risk of illness or injury. Owing to the level of risk associated with class III devices, the FDA has determined that general and special controls alone are insufficient to ensure the safety and effectiveness of class III devices. PMA is the most stringent type of device marketing application required by the FDA. The applicant must receive FDA approval of its PMA application prior to marketing the device. PMA is based on a determination by the FDA that the PMA contains sufficient valid scientific evidence to ensure that the device is safe and effective for its intended use(s).

An approved investigational device exemption (IDE) allows an investigational device to be shipped for the purpose of conducting a clinical study to evaluate the safety and effectiveness of the device. Such data may be used to support a PMA application or a premarket notification [510(k)] submission to the FDA. Most PMA applications contain clinical study data. Only a small percentage of 510(k)s require clinical data to support the application. Investigational use also includes clinical evaluation of certain device modifications or new intended uses of legally marketed devices. All clinical evaluations of investigational devices, unless exempt, must have an approved IDE before the study is initiated. Clinical studies of devices that have not been cleared for marketing require an IDE approved by an institutional review board (IRB). If the study involves a significant risk device, the IDE must also be approved by the FDA.

One specific aim of the Food and Drug Administration Modernization Act of 1997 (FDAMA) is to ensure the timely availability of safe and effective new devices that will benefit the public. One key feature of the FDAMA is the concept of using the least burdensome approach to regulating devices. The CDRH has defined least burdensome as a successful means of addressing a premarket issue that involves the most appropriate investment of time, effort, and resources on the part of industry and the FDA. It is important to note that the statutory thresholds for substantial equivalence or reasonable assurance of safety and effectiveness were not changed by the addition of the least burdensome provisions of the Food, Drug, and Cosmetic Act. More information on the least burdensome approach can be found in "The Least Burdensome Provisions of the FDA Modernization Act of 1997: Concept and Principles," which is available at <http://www.fda.gov/cdrh/ode/guidance/1332.pdf>.

COMBINATION PRODUCTS

Medical devices are regulated in the CDRH, medical drugs are regulated in the Center for Drugs Evaluation and Research (CDER), and medical biologics are regulated in the Center for Biologics Evaluation and Research (CBER). A subset of products requiring premarket review include products that are combinations of a device, drug, or biologic.

The regulation on combination products, 21 CFR Part 3.7, defines these products and discusses the appropriate regulatory approaches. Combination products are increasingly incorporating cutting-edge, novel technologies, and the FDA has been reviewing significantly more combination products as technologic advances continue to merge therapeutic products and blur the historical lines of separation between the FDA's medical product centers. Because combination products involve components that would normally be regulated under different types of regulatory authorities and frequently by different FDA centers, they also raise challenging regulatory, policy, and review management issues. To address these concerns, the FDA's Office of Combination Products was established on December 24, 2002, as required by the Medical Device User Fee and Modernization Act of 2002. The law gives the office broad responsibilities covering the regulatory life cycle of drug-device, drug-biologic, and device-biologic combination products. For more information on the Office of Combination Products, visit their Web page at <http://www.fda.gov/oc/combination>.

Currently, tissue adhesives are regulated in both the CDRH and the CBER, with the lead center for product review currently determined by the primary mode of action of the product.

RESEARCH, IDEs, AND PROTECTION OF HUMAN SUBJECTS

Clinical evaluation of medical devices that have not been cleared for marketing are required to be in compliance with the IDE regulations and approved by an IRB. If the study involves a significant risk device, the FDA must also approve the IDE. Significant risk devices include implants; devices that support or sustain human life; devices that are substantially important in diagnosing, curing, mitigating, or treating disease or in preventing impairment to human health; or devices that present a potential for serious risk to the patient.

The information that needs to be provided in an IDE application can be found at 21 CFR 812.20 or on the FDA's Web site at <www.fda.gov/cdrh/devadvice/ide/index.shtml>. The key elements include a complete description of the device, a report of prior pre-clinical and clinical investigations, the proposed investigational plan, and an informed consent form. The agency strongly encourages anyone who plans to submit an IDE to contact the appropriate reviewing division prior to submitting the IDE.

The FDA recognizes that there may be situations in which the use of an investigational device falls outside the scope of an approved IDE, and yet the use of the investigational device may be the most appropriate option for a particular patient. Depending on the circumstances, emergency use or compassionate use procedures may apply.

Emergency Use

Emergency situations may arise in which there will be a need to use an investigational device in a manner inconsistent with the approved investigational plan or by a physician who is not part of the clinical study. This may occur either before or after the initiation of a clinical trial. The device must be used to treat a life-threatening or serious disease or condition for which there is no alternative, and circumstances should be such that there is no time to obtain FDA approval. Following the emergency use of the device, a follow-up report should be submitted to the FDA in which summary information regarding patient outcome is presented.

Compassionate Use

The compassionate use provision allows access for patients who do not meet the requirements for inclusion in the clinical investigation but for whom the treating physician believes that the device may provide a benefit in treating and/or diagnosing their disease or condition. This provision is typically approved for individual patients but may be approved to treat a small group. The compassionate provisions may apply either during or before a clinical trial is initiated for serious diseases or conditions for which there is no alternative. In both cases, prior FDA approval is needed.

OFF-LABEL USE OF A LEGALLY MARKETED DEVICE

FDA approval of a medical device is, in fact, a decision on both the technology or design of the device itself and its intended use, that is, labeling. Good medical practice and the best interests of the patient require that physicians use legally marketed devices according to their best knowledge and judgment. If physicians use a product for an indication not in the approved labeling, they have the responsibility to be well informed about the device, to base its use on firm scientific rationale and sound medical evidence, and to maintain records of the product's use and effects. Use of a marketed device in this manner when the intent is the "practice of medicine" does not require the submission of an IDE or review by an IRB. However, the institution at which the product will be used may, under its own authority, require IRB review or other institutional oversight. The FDA information sheet on off-label use has additional information and can be found at <http://www.fda.gov/oc/ohrt/irbs/offlabel.html>.

MEDICAL DEVICE REPORTING

Through the premarket review process, the FDA provides reasonable assurance that medical devices are safe and effective for their intended use. Once the device is available for commercial distribution, it is subject to more widespread use. Medical device reporting is the mechanism for the FDA to receive significant medical device adverse events from manufacturers, importers, and user facilities so that they can be detected and corrected quickly.

MedWatch, the FDA Safety Information and Adverse Event Reporting Program, serves both health care professionals and the medical product–using public. The program provides important and timely clinical information about safety issues involving medical products, including prescription and over-the-counter drugs, biologics, dietary supplements, and medical devices. This includes medical product safety alerts, recalls, withdrawals, and important labeling changes that may affect the health of all Americans.

User facilities (eg, hospitals, nursing homes) are required to report suspected medical device–related deaths to both the FDA and the manufacturers. User facilities report medical device–related serious injuries only to the manufacturer. These reports must be made on the MedWatch 3500A Mandatory Reporting Form. In addition, Med-Watch allows health care professionals and consumers to report serious problems that they suspect are associated with the drugs and medical devices they prescribe, dispense, or use. Reporting can be done on-line, by telephone, or by submitting the MedWatch 3500 form by mail or fax.

APPROVED TISSUE ADHESIVE MEDICAL DEVICES

At the present time, only a few tissue adhesive medical devices have received a PMA for use in the United States. The FDA has approved two topical tissue adhesives for soft tissue approximation, Dermabond (2-octyl cyanoacrylate; Closure Medical Corporation, Raleigh, NC) and Indermil (n-butyl-2 cyanoacrylate; United States Surgical Corporation, a Division of Tyco Healthcare Group, LP, Norwalk, CT). Both are indicated for topical application to hold closed thoroughly cleansed, easily approximated skin edges. Two other tissue adhesive medical devices are intended for cardiovascular surgery. BioGlue Surgical Adhesive (Cryolife, Inc., Kennesaw, GA) is made from bovine serum albumin and glutaraldehyde and is indicated for use as an adjunct to standard methods (such as sutures and staples) in adult patients in open surgical repair of large vessels (such as aorta, femoral, and carotid arteries). CoSeal Surgical Sealant (Cohesion Technologies, Inc./Baxter Healthcare International, Palo Alto, CA) is made of two polyethylene glycols, which are mixed together as they are applied to form a glue-like product. CoSeal is indicated for use in vascular reconstructions to achieve adjunctive hemostasis by mechanically sealing areas of leakage.

Anyone wishing to conduct a clinical study of a tissue adhesive for soft tissue approximation must comply with the IDE regulations. This includes clinical investigators who are collecting clinical data for research or other purposes not related to a marketing application. Companies seeking to obtain marketing approval for a new tissue adhesive will need to submit a PMA application and supporting clinical data demonstrating reasonable assurance of the safety and effectiveness of the device when used according to its labeling, that is, indications, contraindications, warnings, and precautions.

Conclusions

Among the future challenges for the FDA with regard to the regulatory oversight of tissue adhesives are the continued development of science-based rationales for regulatory decision-making that will provide a roadmap not only for FDA reviewers but also for industry and the medical community. Such an approach will continue to enhance product review and address questions for manufacturers early on in product development. National and international standards for the manufacture and testing of these products and FDA guidance may be very important.

The CDRH will continue to use different approaches in the science-based, premarket review and postmarket surveillance of tissue adhesive products. These approaches include research, data and information monitoring, postmarket surveillance, regulatory guidance and standards development, training and education for both FDA staff and the research and development community (publications, FDA staff colleges, workshops and conferences), and cooperation with public and private groups.

Continued cooperation and communication between the public and private sector are encouraged so that safe and effective products can reach the public as quickly as possible. The FDA regulatory process for all products, including tissue adhesive products, will continue to be based on product-by-product review, and the agency's science-based approach will continue to provide the information necessary for effective decision-making. As the clinical application of tissue adhesive products evolves, additional issues of product safety and effectiveness will be addressed by the agency as part of its continuing review and assessment of these products.

8 US Food and Drug Administration Perspective on Class I, II, and III Cyanoacrylate Medical Devices

GEORGE J. MATTAMAL, PhD

REGULATORY HISTORY OF DEVICES ASSOCIATED WITH CYANOACRYLATES

The US Food and Drug Administration (FDA) has approved and/or cleared a number of synthetic cyanoacrylates as medical devices since the Medical Device Amendments of 1976 were enacted (see Chapter 7, "US Food and Drug Administration Perspective on the Regulation of Medical Device Tissue Adhesives"). The enactment of the 1976 amendments has expanded the role of the FDA in the regulation of medical devices. The devices are regulated[1] as class I (general controls; with and without exemptions), class II (general and special controls), and class III (general controls and premarket approval [PMA]). The classes to which devices are assigned determine the type of premarketing submission or application required for FDA clearance or approval before marketing. If the device is classified as class I or II and if it is not exempt, a premarket notification [510(k)] will be required. For class III devices, a PMA application will be required. Device classification[1] is assigned based on its intended use and indications for use. Furthermore, classification is risk based, that is, the risk the device poses to the patient and/or the user is a major factor in how a device is classified. Class I includes devices with the lowest risk, and class III includes those with the greatest risk.

How Does the FDA Evaluate Class III Cyanoacrylate Devices for Marketing?

The FDA considers tissue adhesives as "transitional devices," and they are automatically classified as class III devices by the Center for Devices and Radiological Health (CDRH), requiring PMA (see Chapter 7).* The CDRH is one of six centers within the FDA; the other centers are the Center for Drug Evaluation and Research (CDER), the Center for Biologics Evaluation and Research (CBER), the Center for Food Safety and Applied Nutrition (CFSAN), the Center for Veterinary Medicine (CVM), and the National Center for Toxicology Research (NCTR). At the CDRH's Office of Device Evaluation (ODE), manufacturers present the preclinical, clinical, and labeling information that is required for a PMA[2] or product development protocol (see Chapter 2, "History and Background") application for synthetic cyanoacrylate class III devices. Because tissue adhesives are class III devices, they require extensive testing and evaluation for such "high-risk devices." This would include submission of valid scientific evidence to demonstrate reasonable assurance of safety and effectiveness, including laboratory, animal, and clinical data; clinical trials; panel review; and a preapproval inspection. It should be noted that clinical evaluation of "significant risk devices" such as tissue adhesives requires an approved investigational device exemption (IDE)[3] application in addition to institutional review board (IRB) approval.

As explained in Chapter 2, on August 26, 1998, the FDA approved the first class III transitional cyanoacrylate tissue adhesive device for

---

*Transitional devices were regulated previously by the Center for Drugs, Evaluation, and Research (CDER) as new drugs or antibiotic drugs prior to the enactment of the Medical Device Amendments of 1976. Specifically, tissue adhesives and absorbable hemostatic agent and dressing devices were transferred to the CDRH after President Ford signed the Medical Device Amendments to the Food, Drug and Cosmetic Act in 1976.

topical skin approximation, Dermabond (Closure Medical Corporation, Raleigh, NC). It is formulated of over 90% 2-octyl-cyanoacrylate monomer. Following this approval, two other class III cyanoacrylate devices were approved by the FDA. These included the first class III neurologic embolization device formulated with n-butyl-2-cyanoacrylate monomer, Trufill n-Butyl Cyanoacrylate (n-BCA) Liquid Embolic System (Cordis Neurovascular, Inc., Miami Lakes, FL), which was approved on September 25, 2000. It consists of n-butyl-cyanoacrylate (n-BCA), ethiodized oil, and tantalum powder. On May 22, 2002, the FDA approved the second cyanoacrylate tissue adhesive for topical skin approximation, Indermil Tissue Adhesive (United States Surgical, a Division of Tyco Healthcare Group, L.P., Norwalk, CT). It is formulated of over 90% n-butyl-2-cyanoacrylate monomer. Aside from these class III cyanoacrylate devices that were approved via PMA, the FDA cleared via the premarket notification process [510(k)] many class I cyanoacrylate devices (exempt or not exempt) and class II cyanoacrylate devices, such as dental cements and orthodontic bracket adhesives.

HOW DOES THE FDA EVALUATE CLASS I AND II CYANOACRYLATE DEVICES FOR MARKETING?

Medical devices formulated with a major component of cyanoacrylate monomers (alkyl-2-cyanoacrylates) are evaluated at the ODE of the CDRH. The ODE is one of six offices within the CDRH; the other offices are as follows:

- Office of Surveillance and Biometrics (OSB), which monitors devices already on the market
- Office of In Vitro Diagnostics (OIVD), which serves as the primary source for scientific and medical expertise on in vitro diagnostic devices with regard to safety and effectiveness
- Office of Compliance (OC), which acts against firms that violate the law
- Office of Communication, Education and Radiation Programs (OCER), which communicates and educates professionals and consumers on the safe use of devices
- Office of Science and Engineering Laboratories (OSEL), which performs research on device problems

Manufacturers submit premarket notification process [510(k)] submissions[4] containing scientific data in support of class I and II cyanoacrylate devices. These submissions are evaluated at the ODE by ensuring that the medical devices are substantially equivalent to legally marketed devices and are properly manufactured with truthful labeling of the products. Class I and II devices are classified according to risk. For example, class I devices are simple and will have the lowest risk, with a well-established history of safety and effectiveness (ie, general controls), and often may be exempt from premarket notification [510(k)]. Class II devices are generally more complex, will have a moderate risk, and will be required to meet "special controls," such as guidance documents containing the FDA's recommendations, performance standards, postmarket surveillance, tracking requirements, labeling, and sometimes clinical data. Accordingly, for these class II devices (and sometimes class I), the manufacturers submit premarket notification [510(k)] submissions[4] and must show that their devices are substantially equivalent to legally marketed devices in terms of intended use, design configuration, technologic characteristics (or different characteristics but no new safety or effectiveness concerns), function, application, and performance. Information on preparing a 510(k) submission for manufacturers may be found at <http://www.fda.gov/cdrh/devadvice/314.html>.

Class I Cyanoacrylate Devices

The FDA has cleared a few devices associated with cyanoacrylate monomers (alky-2-cyanoacrylates) as class I devices (exempt or not exempt) under product code 79 KMF, Liquid Bandage. Under regulation 21 CFR § 880.5090, a liquid bandage is defined as follows:

(a) *Identification.* A liquid bandage is a sterile device that is a liquid, semiliquid, or powder and liquid combination used to cover an opening in skin or as a dressing for burns. The device is also used as a topical skin protectant.

(b) *Classification.* Class I (general controls). When used only as a skin protectant, the device is exempt from the premarket notification procedures in subpart E of part 807 of this chapter subject to 21 CFR 880. 5090.

The FDA cleared the following class I exempt devices in which the main component of the device was cyanoacrylate monomers (alkyl-2-cyanoacrylates):

1. Superskin Skin Protectant (K972081) (Medlogic Global Corporation, Colorado) was cleared on December 17, 1997. The main component of the device is an alkyl 2-cyanoacrylate monomer. The intended use of the device is "to protect skin exposed to irritation from moisture such as sweat, urine, and digestive juices. It can also be used on unbroken surfaces that are exposed to friction and shear. Do not apply over broken skin." This device is a topically applied skin protectant for use on unbroken skin. The patient applies between two to four drops to the intact skin, and the liquid monomer polymerizes to form a thin, flexible coating.

2. Liquid Bandage (K984192) (GluStitch Inc., Subsidiary of Backlock Medical Products, Inc., British Columbia, Canada) was cleared on February 19, 1999. The main component of the device is n-butyl-2-cyanoacrylate monomer. Indications for use of the device are that it "helps to protect skin exposed to irritation from moisture such as sweat, urine, and digestive juices. It can also be used on unbroken surfaces that are exposed to friction and shear. Do not apply over broken skin."

These class I (exempt) devices with the major component of cyanoacrylate monomers (alkyl-2-cyanoacrylates) may be available for over-the-counter (OTC) use by consumers.

Also, the FDA cleared the following class 1 (not exempt) devices in which the major component was cyanoacrylate monomers (alkyl-2-cyanoacrylates):

1. Liquiderm Liquid Adhesive Bandage (K002338) (Closure Medical Corporation) was cleared on January 29, 2001. It is a sterile, clear, free-flowing liquid containing D&C violet #2 and an antimicrobial preservation system to prevent contamination on repeated opening of the primary container. The main component of the device is 2-octyl cyanoacrylate monomer. LiquidermLiquid Adhesive Bandage is intended for OTC use "to cover minor cuts, scrapes, burns, and minor irritations of the skin and help protect them from infection."

2. LiquiShield-S (K023163) (MedLogic Global Limited, Plymouth, UK) was cleared on January 13, 2003. The main component of the device is a cyanoacrylate monomer (alkyl-2-cyanoacrylate), and its applicator and packaging are sterilized. It is applied as a liquid and dries within 45 seconds, adhering to the contours of skin to form a transparent flexible film. LiquiShield-S is intended "to protect intact or damaged skin from the effects of moisture, friction (rubbing), or shear (tearing). It helps protect skin exposed

to irritation from moisture such as urine, faeces, digestive juices, perspiration and wound drainage. It can also be used in areas that are exposed to friction and shear such as occurs when items, such as bedding, clothing, or shoes, rub against the skin. LiquiShield-S helps protect the skin against irritation caused by adhesive products."

3. GluSeal (K030574) (GluStitch, Inc.) was cleared on August 21, 2003. The main component of the device is 2-octyl cyanoacrylate monomer. It is intended "to cover minor cuts, scrapes, burns, and minor irritations of the skin and help protect them from infection."

4. 3M Liquid Bandage (K031263) (3M Health Care, St. Paul, MN) was cleared on October 21, 2003. It is a sterile, clear, n-2-butyl cyanoacrylate liquid that is packaged in an aluminum tube with a reusable cap. 3M Liquid Bandage is indicated for use as an OTC device for consumers "to cover minor cuts, scrapes, and skin irritations."

5. LiquidShield Liquid Bandage (K031321) (MedLogic Global Limited) was cleared on January 21, 2004. The main component of the device is cyanoacrylate monomers (alkyl-2-cyanoacrylates), and its applicator and packaging are sterilized. It is applied as a liquid, which, on contact with the skin, dries within 45 seconds, adhering to the contours of skin to form a transparent flexible film. It wears off naturally as the skin regenerates. LiquiShield Liquid Bandage is intended for OTC use "to cover minor cuts and scrapes and minor irritations of the skin and help protect them from infection."

Class II Cyanoacrylate Devices

The FDA has cleared a number of class II dental cements and orthodontic bracket adhesives in which the major component was cyanoacrylate monomers (alkyl-2-cyanoacrylates).

Class II Dental Cements Containing Cyanoacrylates

Dental cements containing cyanoacrylates are categorized with product code 76 EMA (cement, dental), and these devices are class II based on 21 CFR § 872.3275. Under this regulation, dental cement is defined as follows:

(b) Dental cement other than zinc oxide-eugenol
(1) *Identification.* Dental cement other than zinc oxide-eugenol is a device composed of various materials other than zinc

oxide-eugenol intended to serve as a temporary tooth filling or as a base cement to affix dental devices such as crowns or bridges, or to be applied to a tooth to protect the tooth pulp. (2) *Classification.* Class II.

The FDA cleared the following dental cement class I devices in which the major component was cyanoacrylate monomers (alkyl-2-cyanoacrylates):

1. GluSite (K013446) (GluStitch) was cleared on December 20, 2001. It contains 2-octyl cyanoacrylate monomer (a major component) and is a clear, colorless, free-flowing liquid monomer packaged in glass multiple-use vials. On contact with weak bases, GluSite polymerizes to form a strong adhesive bond. GluSite is intended for use "as dental cement for bonding dental materials such as crowns, caps, and pins, or temporarily attaching a fiber to the surface of tooth in a procedure to treat periodontal disease."

2. Liquidband Dental (K993556) (MedLogic Global Corporation) was cleared on January 3, 2000. The major component of the device is n-butyl cyanoacrylate, which is a clear, colorless, free-flowing liquid packaged in a single-use, 0.5 g, high-density polyethylene ampule with an attachable polypropylene applicator tip. On seating the cap or crown and contact with weak bases, Liquidband Dental polymerizes as it forms a strong adhesive between the cap or crown and the tooth. It is intended for use "as an adhesive when bonding of caps and crowns to teeth is required."

3. Periacryl (K974097) (Blacklock Medical Products, Inc., British Columbia, Canada) was cleared on April 9, 1998. The major component of the device is n-butyl 2-cyanoacrylate monomer. The device is indicated for use "as a dental cement for bonding dental materials such as crowns, caps, and pins."

4. Indermil Dental (K960910) (Loctite Corporation, Connecticut) was cleared on March 28, 1996. It is a liquid n-butyl 2-cyanoacrylate monomer that cures in the presence of anions. It is sterilized by gamma radiation and is provided for use in high-density polyethylene dispensers. The device is indicated for use "as a dental cement for bonding dental materials, such as crowns, caps, and pins; or temporarily attaching a fiber to the surface of the tooth in a procedure to treat periodontal disease."

5. Cyanodont Dental Cement (K901082) (Specialites Septodent, Washington, DC) was cleared on July 9, 1990. The major component of the device is n-butyl 2- cyanoacrylate monomer. The device is indicated for use "as a dental cement in cementation of dental prostheses."

6. Octyldent (K884652) (CRX Medical, Inc., North Carolina) was cleared on May 24, 1989. The major component of the device is 2-octyl cyanoacrylate monomer. The device is intended for use "as an adhesive when bonding of crown and caps to teeth is desired."

7. Octyldent (2-octyl cyanoacrylate) (K980159) (Closure Medical Corporation) was cleared on April 9, 1998. The major component of the device is 2-octyl cyanoacrylate monomer. The device is intended for use "as an adhesive for the temporary fixing of periodontal polymer or fibers in periodontal pockets."

8. Additional Indication for Octyldent (K902078) (2-octyl cyanoacrylate) (CRX Medical) was cleared on August 3, 1990. The major component of the device is 2-octyl cyanoacrylate monomer. The device is intended to be used to "to adhere fibers impregnated with tetracycline antibiotic to teeth."

9. Nexadent (K870209) (Bionexus, Inc., North Carolina) was cleared on February 19, 1987. The major component of the device is n-butyl 2-cyanoacrylate monomer. The device is intended for use as a dental cement.

10. Cyanobond (K770067) (Parkell Products, Inc., New York) was cleared on January 23, 1977. The major component of the device is either ethyl-2-cyanoacrylate or n-propyl-2-cyanoacrylate or n-butyl-2-cyanoacrylate monomer. The device is intended for use as "a dental cementing medium to cement dental pins and posts; to repair and cement fractured porcelain and acrylic crowns and teeth; to repair broken dentures and stone models."

11. Iso-Dent (Ellman International Manufacturing, Hewlett, NY) is a preamendment device marketed prior to 1976. It should be noted that prior to the 1976 amendments, the FDA did not regulate medical devices. The major component of the device is isobutyl-2-cyanoacrylate monomer. The device is intended for use as a dental cement.

Certain class II dental cements containing cyanoacrylates are categorized with product code 76 MZW (dental cement without zinc oxide–eugenol as ulcer covering), and these devices are class II based on 21 CFR § 872.3275.

Soothe-N-Seal Canker Sore Relief (K991923) (Closure Medical, Corporation) was cleared on September 2, 1999. The device is composed of over 99% of 2-octyl cyanoacrylate monomer. It polymerizes to form a thin, protective film, typically within 5 seconds. Once polymerized, the applied layer of 2-octyl cyanoacrylate has a high degree of adhesion strength and flexibility. The film remains adhered to the tissue surface until the underlying tissue to which it is bonded is spontaneously sloughed through natural reepithelialization or until mechanically displaced. It is a non-sterile, clear, colorless, free-flowing liquid protectant packaged in high-density, polyethylene, multiple-use, controlled dropper bottles. The device package contains 1 g of liquid protectant and 10 double-ended applicator swabs in a transparent polyethylene terephthalate tray with a cardboard display label. Each end of the swab handle consists of a polyurethane foam sponge tip, with one end rounded for drying the ulcer area and one end pointed for device application.

Closure Medical Corporation performed two clinical studies to demonstrate the safety and effectiveness of Soothe-N-Seal Canker Sore Relief in the management of oral ulcers. The first clinical study was a single-center study of 42 subjects who were randomized to treatment with one of the two device formulations or to sham treatment using saline. The second clinical study was a multicenter clinical study of 155 subjects who were randomized to receive either the subject device (Soothe-N-Seal Canker Sore Relief), a predicate device (the Carrington OraPatch) such as K933741, K964852, or a negative control (water). The intended use of Soothe-N-Seal Canker Sore Relief is to create "a thin, protective barrier that provides relief of pain associated with canker sores, mouth sores, and traumatic ulcers, such as those caused by braces."

Class II Orthodontic Bracket Adhesives Containing Cyanoacrylates

Orthodontic bracket adhesives containing cyanoacrylates are categorized with product code 76 DYH (adhesive, bracket and tooth conditioner, resin) and are class II based on 21 CFR § 872.3750. Under this regulation, bracket adhesive resin and tooth conditioner are defined as follows:

> (a) Identification. A bracket adhesive resin and tooth conditioner is a device composed of an adhesive compound, such as polymethylmethacrylate, intended to cement an orthodontic bracket to a tooth surface.
> (b) Classification. Class II.

The FDA cleared the following class II orthodontic bracket adhesives, which consist mainly of cyanoacrylate monomers (alkyl-2-cyanoacrylates):

1. Smart-Bond (K981036) (G.A.C. International, Inc., New York) was cleared on April 5, 1999. The main component of the device is an alkyl 2-cyanoacrylate monomer. The indication of use is "as an orthodontic bonding agent, for the bonding of orthodontic braces on the tooth (brackets, tubes, and which adhere of) for a limited period of time."

2. Gridlock 195 (Allodex Systems, Arizona) was cleared on May 1, 2002. The main component of the device is an alkyl 2-cyanoacrylate monomer. The indication for use of the device is for cementing orthodontic brackets to teeth.

SUMMARY

As explained in this chapter, since 1976, the FDA has approved and/or cleared a number of class I, II, and III cyanoacrylate medical devices in which the main component is a cyanoacrylate homolog. Because of the distinct differences in the properties of various cyanoacrylate homologs and their formulations, these devices should be used appropriately as class I, II, or III devices, depending on their clinical applications, labeling, and indications for use. Currently, many cyanoacrylate medical devices of various regulatory classes are under review by the FDA.

REFERENCES

1. US Food and Drug Administration. Classify your medical device. Available at: http://www.fda.gov/cdrh/devadvice/313.html (accessed Oct 14, 2004).

2. US Food and Drug Administration. Overview of premarket approval (PMA). Available at: http://www.fda.gov/cdrh/devadvice/pma/ (accessed Oct 14, 2004).

3. US Food and Drug Administration. Overview of investigational device exemption (IDE). Available at: http://www.fda.gov/crdh/devadvice/ide/index.shtml.

4. US Food and Drug Administration. Premarket notification [510(k)]. Available at: http://www.fda.gov/cdrh/devadvice/314.html.

Index